ABOUT TH

Jon Sandifer began to travel and work his way around the world at the age of 17. During his six years of travels through 52 countries, he developed a growing interest in Oriental philosophy and healing systems. At the age of 23 he began to eat macrobiotic food and enrolled at the Kushi Institute in London to train as a macrobiotic teacher and counsellor. Initially he studied the work of Michio Kushi, which involved learning macrobiotic cookery, macrobiotic medicine, Oriental diagnosis, Yin and Yang, Shiatsu massage and the Japanese exercise routine Do-In. He also took up the Japanese martial art Aikido and learnt the basics of anatomy, physiology and nutrition.

He began teaching macrobiotics and started to develop the curriculum of the Kushi Institute in London, liaising with other institutes in the USA and Europe. Over the next decade he taught all over the world and counselled thousands of individuals on macrobiotics. In recent years he has developed his interest in Feng Shui. He currently chairs the Feng Shui Society (UK) and continues to write on the subject. Macrobiotics, for him, is Inner Feng Shui, as he appreciates the importance of working in harmony with our inner and outer worlds.

He is the author of several books including *A Piatkus Guide to Feng Shui* (1999), *Feng Shui Journey* (1999) and *Feng Shui Astrology* (1997), all published by Piatkus, *The 10-Day Re-balance Programme* (Rider Books, 1997) and *Acupressure* (Element Books, 1997).

In addition to his work and studies, he has been blessed with seven healthy children.

DEDICATION

To the unsung heroines of macrobiotics whose cookery classes or lectures have inspired me and countless others through their skill and dedication: Ann Duggan, Anna Ledvinka, Anna Mackenzie, Anne Dreschler, Annie Tara, Aveline Kushi, Cornelia Aihara, Daphne Watson, Dawn Gilmour, Eugenia Varatojo, Françoise Riviere, Geraldine Walker, Gosia Gorna, Jan Snyder, Jean Cox, Joannie Spear, Judy Waxman, Karen Acuff, Kathleen Burns, Kristina Turner, Lesley Willis, Lima Ohsawa, Linda Burn, Maria Gillet, Marion Price, Marion Sandifer, Marilyn Waxman, Marlise Binneti, Melanie Waxman, Mieke Vervecken-Pieters, Montse Bradford, Pam Snyder, Renata Sandifer, Shirley Roach, Shizuko Yamamoto, Susie Caunce, Susan Krieger, Susan O'Toole, Weike Nelissen and Wendy Esko.

Macrobiotics
FOR BEGINNERS

Macrobiotics
FOR BEGINNERS

*How to achieve
health and vitality
the Oriental way*

JON SANDIFER

With recipes by Bob Lloyd

PIATKUS

Published in the UK in 2000 by
Judy Piatkus (Publishers) Limited
5 Windmill Street
London W1P 1HF
e-mail: info@piatkus.co.uk

For the latest news and information on all our titles, visit
our website at www.piatkus.co.uk

A catalogue record for this book is available from the British Library

ISBN 0-7499-2119-6

Design by Paul Saunders
Edited by Kelly Davis

Typeset by Action Publishing Technology Ltd, Gloucester
Printed and bound in Great Britain by Biddles Ltd, Guildford
www.biddles.co.uk

CONTENTS

ACKNOWLEDGEMENTS

My thanks to Michio and Aveline Kushi for their untiring work these past 50 years in the West; for their writing, their teaching and their endless energy in pursuit of their dream of one peaceful world. To Bob Lloyd for all the effort he put into creating the wonderful recipes in this book and for his dedication as current Chairman of the Macrobiotic Association of Great Britain. To my sister, Mary, for typing and preparing the whole manuscript – thank you. To my wife, Renata, for sustaining me with her delicious and inspiring food.

INTRODUCTION

In this modern age we are all united by our desire for good health, good relationships with others and financial stability. The most important of these three factors is our health, as it underpins the other two. Macrobiotics offers an all-embracing approach to good health, as it encompasses diet, lifestyle and traditional wisdom. Diet is the most fundamental aspect and, by following a macrobiotic diet, we can gain far more control over our health.

In order to restore balance and harmony in our bodies without recourse to expensive treatment or medicine, we need something we can put into practice ourselves. The first step in macrobiotics is to return to using simple, traditional foods. As human beings, we have evolved over thousands of years and the modern diet can be a challenge to our system. (Rather like a motor vehicle, if we service it regularly and use the appropriate fuel, it will run efficiently and smoothly.) The second step, lifestyle, is to get back in touch with the basic disciplines that our ancestors practised instinctively, such as rising early, not eating before sleeping, chewing food very well, and taking exercise every day. The third step is to acknowledge and remember the universal truth asserted by ancient spiritual teachers – that we are ultimately responsible for our lives. Once you truly accept that you are responsible for your own health, and undertake a lifestyle that supports and motivates your body and soul (fuelling your system in a way that is appropriate for your individual needs), then you will access new levels of health and vitality.

The benefits can be enormous. Over the past 20 years I have witnessed extraordinary changes, not only in my own health but in that of my clients, students and associates. They include:

♦ greater stamina

♦ a bigger appetite for life

♦ sharper memory

♦ greater alertness

♦ emotional stability

♦ physical flexibility

♦ increased sensitivity

♦ regained intuition

♦ a new spiritual awareness

- ♦ a greater sense of freedom

- ♦ recovery from disease

- ♦ prevention of disease

- ♦ stronger immune system

- ♦ more adaptable behaviour

These are only some of the benefits that thousands of people have achieved by following the macrobiotic path, and it is important and inspiring to remember that they did this themselves! Unlike some other approaches to healing, where the work is done for you, here *you* take the helm – and that in itself is both rewarding and educational.

HOW TO USE THIS BOOK

In this book, based on over 20 years' experience practising macrobiotics, teaching future counsellors and advising those with health problems, I have covered what I consider to be the essence of this broad and fascinating subject.

Chapter 1 explains the origins of macrobiotics and how it has developed, and Chapters 2 to 5 introduce you to the underlying principles, including an overview of the universal and dynamic relationship of Yin and Yang, the seven levels of health, how the food you eat affects your health, and how you can begin to eliminate toxins from your system.

In Chapter 6, using Oriental diagnosis and Yin and Yang principles, I show you how to assess your current health status. You will be able to refer back to this section over the years and adjust your diet as your condition changes. Chapter 7 outlines all the ingredients used in the macrobiotic diet and the principles that have been central to all cooking preparation over the past several thousand years.

In Chapter 8, Bob Lloyd (Chairman of the Macrobiotic Association) contributes an excellent selection of macrobiotic recipes to get you started. There are ideas for breakfast, lunch, supper and snacks.

Chapter 9 explains the suggestions for a macrobiotic lifestyle, including advice on exercise and other aspects of daily life that can enhance your health.

Finally, Chapter 10 and the resource lists at the back of the book explain where you can find a macrobiotic cookery teacher or counsellor, where to buy these foods and how to network with other macrobiotic people.

1

THE BEGINNINGS OF MACROBIOTICS

The term 'macrobiotics' was coined by the Japanese writer and teacher George Ohsawa in the 1940s, from the Greek 'macro' (meaning 'big') and 'bios' (life) – the big life. Drawing on his own personal experience and eclectic study of both Western and Eastern spiritual teachings, Ohsawa encouraged a return to simple foods, natural ingredients, and locally grown seasonal foods – in response to the rapid changes that were taking place in agricultural policy at that time. In many ways, Ohsawa was years ahead of his time, as people are now far more aware of the dangers of genetically modified foods, pesticides, herbicides and artificial growing techniques.

THE MODERN PIONEERS

In more recent times, macrobiotics has been developed by several former students of Ohsawa, including Michio and Aveline Kushi who established themselves in Boston, Massachusetts, in 1960.

From humble beginnings (teaching cookery and supplying basic macrobiotic ingredients from the basement of their home), they soon developed a school and a store, and gained an increasing reputation in the 1970s. Michio and Aveline Kushi were responsible for developing the Kushi Institute – a teacher training programme for macrobiotic practitioners in the US with affiliates in Europe. They also established what is now one of the largest chains of natural food stores – Erewhon Foods – and the natural health magazine, the *East West Journal*.

Meanwhile, in California, Cornelia and Herman Aihara established the Vega Study Centre where they devoted themselves to teaching Ohsawa's work, translating his books and training future teachers and counsellors. Another former student of Ohsawa's, Tomio Kikuchi, established a centre in Brazil, and he also travels and teaches extensively throughout the world.

Shizuko Yamamoto, another student of Ohsawa's who came to the United States in the early 1960s, established herself in New York and has made an enormous contribution to the development of shiatsu (massage using the acupuncture points) through her teaching and books.

Many of the pioneers of macrobiotics had a background in martial arts and shiatsu. Part of the early studies of macrobiotics in the West included sessions of this massage and palm healing.

MACROBIOTICS TODAY

There are literally thousands of people worldwide who have adopted macrobiotic principles in their daily lives. There are various publications, networks and internet sites, summer camps and schools, details of which I have listed at the back of this book. Macrobiotics has had an impact on many areas of our society, with the growth of interest in organic farming, natural food processing, shiatsu massage, Far Eastern medicine and Feng Shui. The Kushis have inspired many projects that are currently being developed and researched. Here are a few examples:

♦ In Russia, doctors are using macrobiotic foods to help counteract the effects of exposure to nuclear radiation (because of the anti-toxic effects of miso and sea vegetables).

♦ The Kellog School of Management at Northwestern University in Evanston, USA, is serving macrobiotic food in its executive dining room.

♦ The Ritz-Carlton Hotels and the Prince Hotels are serving macrobiotic food in their dining rooms worldwide.

- The Smithsonian Institute in Washington, DC, honoured the Kushis and their work in 1999 by creating archives to store their contribution to the health and diet revolution in the USA.

- Recently the US Department of Agriculture issued national standards for organic foods for the first time. This officially recognises the superiority of chemical-free foods which the Kushis and their associates have actively campaigned for over the past 30 years.

- The National Institute of Health (NIH) is currently researching the macrobiotic approach to cancer through a grant awarded to the University of Minnesota in co-operation with the Kushi Institute.

2

THE WORLD OF YIN AND YANG

◈

The terms Yin and Yang have been used for centuries in Tibet, China, Korea, Japan and Taiwan to describe two opposite yet complementary forces that appear in all natural phenomena. From a Western scientific viewpoint, one might regard Yin and Yang as the polarities of plus and minus, north and south, male and female, night and day, hot and cold, slow and fast, etc.

The principle of Yin and Yang applies both to the food you eat and to your own state or condition. You can therefore learn to determine whether your current condition is more Yin (tired, withdrawn, slow) or more Yang (aggressive, impatient, stubborn) and balance the condition by eating foods that represent the opposite nature. Let's look at a few examples.

Foods that have a cooling or relaxing nature, such as alcoholic beverages, sugar, ice cream and fruits, are usually regarded as more Yin. Because of their Yin nature, such foods would help to balance somebody who was overly Yang – hot or aggressive. In the same way, these Yin foods would help us to combat living in an environment that was excessively Yang (hot, dry or active). This is the major reason why, when you live in the tropics or go on holiday where it is warm, you automatically feel more drawn to relaxing or Yin foods. Conversely, if you are undertaking hard, physical, manual work in the depths of winter (Yin), when it is freezing cold (Yin), then you are going to need the fire, heat and Yang qualities that warmer, more savoury foods will bring.

YIN AND YANG EMOTIONS

To determine how you are feeling at present, look at the following columns of Yin and Yang emotions. If you relate more to one column than the other, then that tells you that you are feeling more Yin or Yang.

Yin	Yang
nervous	inflexible
worried	demanding
introverted	unreasonable
emotional	impatient
lack of concentration	aggressive
indecision	irritable
lack of memory	impulsive

YIN AND YANG FOODS

The next step is to determine what kinds of foods, generally, you need to eat to balance your current condition. We can recognise Yin/Yang foods by their characteristics and the effects they have (see below). If your current condition is more Yin, then you need to introduce qualities of the opposite category (more Yang) into your diet.

Characteristics of Yin foods

higher in potassium

prefer warm or hot climates

grow faster

grow larger

grow taller

softer

watery

grow upwards

grow horizontally below the ground

larger leaves

Characteristics of Yang foods

higher in sodium

prefer cold or cool climates

grow slowly

grow smaller

grow shorter

harder

drier

grow horizontally above the ground

grow vertically below the ground

smaller leaves

Of course, the Yin/Yang nature of a food can be changed by how it is prepared and cooked (see pages 12–16).

Some foods are neither Yin nor Yang and these are

described as 'balanced'. Some examples of typical foods in each category are given below:

Yin foods	Yang foods	Balanced foods
alcohol	salt	grains
sugar	eggs	vegetables
coffee	miso	nuts
tropical fruit	shoyu	seeds
ice cream	red meat	beans
milk	game	sea vegetables (seaweeds)
	poultry	
	fish	

The characteristics of the food determine what effect it will have on us:

The effect of Yin foods	The effect of Yang foods
cooler	warmer
softer	harder
calmer	faster
slower	less sleepy
relaxed	more impatient
	irritable

YIN AND YANG IN COOKING

All cooking, anywhere in the world, is fundamentally based on four factors. These are:

- **fire**: the use and quality of flame

- **time**: how long the food is cooked for

- **pressure**: whether or not we use a lid, an oven or even a pressure cooker

- **salt**: how much, if any, salt is used in the cooking process.

It is really a combination of these four factors that transmutes the raw ingredients into a meal. Essentially, the more you use any of these factors, the more Yang the food becomes. And the less you use these factors (of fire, time, pressure and salt), the more Yin the food becomes.

In this context, the word 'fire' represents flame. The higher the flame, the more Yang the food becomes; and the lower the flame, the softer the cooking style and the more Yin the result. Mellower, sweeter dishes are cooked on a low flame, and foods that have no flame at all – raw – are the most Yin of all. Dishes that require a very high flame, such as tempura (Japanese deep-fried), are regarded as more Yang.

If the cooking time is nil, as in raw foods, then the outcome is more Yin; whereas a dish that takes 3–4 hours to cook is inevitably far more Yang. Practically speaking, quick styles of cooking are more Yin, whereas lengthier styles (such as roasting, baking and casseroling) are regarded as more Yang.

The obvious source of pressure nowadays is the

pressure cooker. Although this is a good cooking method for brown rice and occasionally for bean dishes, it is not recommended for the lighter, softer (more Yin) ingredients such as vegetables. In earlier times, pressure just meant whether the meal was cooked in a heavy pot with a tight-fitting lid or simply cooked inside an oven.

Very salty dishes are naturally far more Yang than those that have little or no salt at all. But it is when you start to combine all four factors that you really see the principles at work. For example, an extremely Yang dish would be one which was cooked on a high flame for a long time, under extreme pressure and that was salty. At the other extreme, a raw dish that was made using no flame, in a short period of time, with no pressure and no salt, would be the ultimate Yin preparation. Between these two extremes lies a whole variety of cooking styles that together make up the art of macrobiotic cuisine.

An example of how you might apply these principles would be in preparing a salmon steak. As an ingredient, fish (and especially salmon) is relatively Yang, so if you were to prepare it with a high flame, for a long time, under pressure and with plenty of salt, it might be totally inappropriate for somebody who is already too Yang. To balance the Yang quality of salmon, it would be better to use a lower flame, to prepare it over a relatively short period of time (15 minutes), with no pressure – steaming or poaching would seem ideal. Finally, only season it modestly with salt or shoyu.

You can see from this example that smoked salmon would be extremely Yang, relative to raw salmon (used in sashimi) which would be the Yin extreme. Instinctively, we know that smoked salmon is very Yang and it is almost always accompanied by liberal amounts of lemon juice, and served thinly sliced on bread to help us avoid eating too much of it. Finally it is often accompanied by a very Yin form of alcohol – champagne.

For easy reference, here is a list of cooking styles, beginning with the most Yin and ending with the most Yang:

Yin
raw
blanching
boiling
steaming
pressing (a quick pickle)
water sauté (to sauté with water instead of oil)
oil sauté
pickling
stir-frying
pressure cooking
baking
deep-frying

Yang

According to traditional wisdom, Yin represents: slower energy, and colder, damper, softer material; whereas Yang represents energy that is faster and material that is warmer, drier, smaller and harder. There's no need to be over-awed by the terms. The fact is that we have all been using Yin/Yang principles subconsciously all our lives. We know that when we have been working too hard we need to take a break, we know that when our food is too savoury we need more fluids, we know that when we are cold we need warmth, and we know that when we are under pressure we need our own space. All these are fundamental examples of Yin and Yang.

3

THE SEVEN LEVELS
OF HEALTH

Many people initially become interested in macrobiotics because they would like to achieve better health. Within a couple of months most of them notice increased levels of energy and vitality and a new-found sensitivity to what their bodies need. However, it is important to understand what health actually means. The following seven levels (or aspects) of health were originally defined by George Ohsawa and later refined by his student and associate, Michio Kushi.

The first four levels are relatively easy and can be achieved in 30 days. The last three levels take longer – for some a few months, but for others one to two years – as the biological effect of food changing the blood impacts on our nervous system and consciousness.

1 NO TIREDNESS

Fatigue has many causes. The usual ones are transitory and are commonly caused by either over-eating, over-sleeping, not exercising enough, or physical or mental stress. This kind of fatigue can quite easily be reversed within a couple of days by reviewing how you are eating, sleeping, exercising and dealing with stress.

It is a very different quality of tiredness from that which we get when we have been working extremely hard or exercising and 'deserve' to feel tired. We have all experienced that kind of tiredness – after a full day's exertion and plenty of fresh air, we are asleep as soon as our head hits the pillow.

However, the other kind of fatigue is much more pervasive. And unless we take action it can soon become chronic, affecting our thinking, our performance and our general interest in life. Many people seem to *expect* that they are going to be tired and therefore limit their capacity to enjoy themselves. How many of us when we receive an invitation on Monday to go to a dinner party on Friday evening, decline it because we expect we will be too 'tired' by then?

If we become chronically tired, then this lack of energy pervades all we do, starting a vicious cycle. Our cooking becomes tired and unenthusiastic, our creativity is dampened, our desire to socialise diminishes, and so on.

Tiredness is the easiest level to reverse using macrobiotics. Because the food is easier to digest people report

feeling lighter and more enthusiastic. Importantly, tiredness is often caused by our thinking – when we engage in
new projects that benefit our health, inevitably we are
charged with new-found enthusiasm.

2 GOOD APPETITE

You must have noticed that the hungriest people in our
society are children! Not only are they constantly
demanding meals and snacks but they are also endlessly
curious (another facet of appetite that is vital to our
health). If chronic tiredness is not quickly reversed, it will
undoubtedly affect our appetite or curiosity about others,
the world around us, our creativity and our dreams. We
have all met fascinating elderly people who maintain
their health, I believe, primarily because of their appetite.
They are curious to find out more about the world they
live in, they take up evening courses, they learn how to
use the internet, they read, they socialise, and they like to
keep abreast of what is new.

Naturally, if we take in too much of anything we
become over-saturated and we lose our appetite. Hence,
one of the recommendations in macrobiotics is to eat
only to 80 per cent of your capacity and to avoid eating
at all if you are not hungry.

3 GOOD SLEEP

Sleep, as we all know, is vital to our health (both mental and physical). However, there is much debate as to how much sleep we actually need. Given that we are all physiologically different and our condition, in terms of Yin and Yang, is constantly changing, the amount we need should reflect this. There are no hard and fast rules but anywhere between six and nine hours a night would appear to be normal.

It is not just the *amount* of sleep but also the *quality* that Ohsawa stressed was important. Good sleep is when you fall asleep immediately without tossing and turning for hours, when you do not have nightmares or night sweats, and your sleep is not disturbed in order to visit the bathroom. Another sign of good sleep is that you wake naturally, without the aid of an alarm clock and not in a state of confusion, wondering what your agenda is for the day or where your clothes are!

As with appetite and curiosity, children are excellent examples of good sleep. They seem to know exactly how much they need. They fall asleep quickly and wake up bright-eyed and eager to take on the day and the world.

4 GOOD MEMORY

There are, I believe, three levels of memory. The first I would call 'mechanical'. This relates to our capacity to remember details such as telephone numbers, shopping lists, our schedule, people's names and what the time is. On some days this mechanical memory works like a charm but on other days we may appear scatty and forgetful.

The second level of memory is 'biological' – the memory that is deeply rooted in every cell, fibre and structure of our physical being. Modern science may like to call this our DNA. From a biological perspective, we never need to remind our lungs to breathe, or our hearts to beat, or our liver to perform its thousand different complex and intricate functions every day. We take all this for granted, but when we become chronically ill, and our health degenerates, what we are really suffering from is a form of biological amnesia. Put simply, the cells in the body have forgotten how to operate. One of the central beliefs in macrobiotics is that if we begin to live and eat in harmony with the way our systems have been designed by evolution, then that biological memory will return and we will regain our health. Certainly, in my time as a macrobiotic counsellor, I have witnessed countless examples of biological memory returning in this way and restoring the person to health.

The third aspect of memory I call 'spiritual'. This is the kind of memory or realisation that we have all experienced from time to time throughout our lives when we feel entirely at one with ourselves and the world in which we live. For me, there were magic moments in my childhood and youth, in my career and in fatherhood that made me realise all was well! And the longer I practise macrobiotics, the more these feelings of being at one with myself, my dream and destiny occur. Having talked to many friends who have had similar experiences, I believe that this is a wonderful and unexpected side-effect of practising macrobiotics. When we regain this memory, we have no fear of the future. Instead, our own ups and downs are set against a far larger picture of time and space. Deep down, we know who we are and where we are. As a result, we always feel 'at home', wherever we are.

5 NEVER ANGRY

According to Ohsawa, the four preceding levels of health are relatively easy to change once you begin to practise macrobiotics. The road gets harder as we work through these next three.

Anger, I believe, is an important emotion to experience from time to time. Simply smiling beatifically, when confronted by a situation that demands swift action, is clearly not the answer. In fact we can harness anger in a very positive way. For example, you may feel very strongly about a political situation, a local environmental issue, or some aspect of the education of your children. In such a case, utilising this emotion of anger creatively can add a lot more force to what you are trying to achieve.

I believe that what Ohsawa possibly meant was 'no resentment'. Resentment is an insidious form of anger that is not healthily released from the system. It builds up within the individual and begins to erode their self-esteem, their vitality, their self-expression and their relationships with others. Having given macrobiotic counselling for many years, I can safely say that unresolved resentment, in my opinion, is a far greater cause of illness than what people eat. It takes a lot of effort, energy and stamina to keep resentment continually stoked up. But, once this resentment has been released, through forgiveness, the individual can find far more positive channels for their energy and creativity.

Essential to the practice of macrobiotics is a sense of humour! The idiosyncrasies of macrobiotic practice, the mistakes we inevitably make when we begin, the strange new cooking ingredients, and the comments of our friends and families, all require a great deal of flexibility and humour to cope with! Oriental wisdom has also advised for centuries that we turn our enemies into our friends. 'Good humour', from the days of Chaucer down to our own time, has always been about flexibility in both body and soul.

6 JOYFUL AND ALERT

There is a strong correlation between the previous five levels of health and the healthy workings of our internal organs. The processes of digestion, absorption and elimination are all reflected in the quality of our blood and how we respond physically and emotionally as a result.

Our capacity to feel joy and to be alert tells us about a different aspect of our internal structure – namely the health and well-being of our nervous system.

From an Oriental perspective, our nervous system is seen as a conductor of energy from Heaven and Earth, and the way we filter and receive this charge corresponds to the way we perceive and respond to the world around us. When our nervous systems becomes tired and dulled, our response naturally declines. Conversely, when our nervous system is clear and sharp, our judgement, wit and response are heightened. Over the past two decades, the idea of 'taking responsibility for our health' has been much in vogue. Interestingly, the word 'responsibility' actually means 'the ability to respond' (respond-ability).

It is this aspect of health – the slow dulling of the individual's nervous system – that concerns me most. If we are over-awed by data, technology, noise and distractions, and at the same time fuel our nervous system with foods that can potentially dull it (animal fats), or foods that over-excite it (refined carbohydrates and stimulants), then it is our individual and collective judgement that is going to pay the price.

A healthy nervous system not only needs to be fuelled appropriately but exercised at the same time. Any kind of racquet sport, martial art or competitive sport, practised regularly, can help keep this system sharp and focused. One thing that continues to amaze me about macrobiotic children is the quality and sharpness of their nervous system. Ohsawa, justifiably, felt that this was represented

best by our capacity to be alert to what was going on
around us and joyful and enthusiastic in all that we took
on.

7 ENDLESS APPRECIATION

This challenging level of health can be summarised
simply as 'having gratitude'. In essence, this means that
whatever trials and tribulations, difficulties and struggles
we experience, we can learn from them and be grateful for
the lessons they teach us. Without a degree of struggle or
challenge, we would rarely learn much. To honestly, and
with integrity, have this kind of appreciation, we need
complete faith in what Ohsawa called 'the Order of the
Universe'.

The opposite quality to appreciation or gratitude is
arrogance. This can take the form of believing that our
struggles are all somebody else's fault, or that we are the
victim. Arrogance can also be shown in not allowing any
self-reflection to occur and simply battling on, regardless
of any change, flexibility or advice that is offered.

4

FUELLING THE BODY – INPUT AND OUTPUT

One of the underlying principles of macrobiotics is that we should be aware of the quality of our daily intake of 'fuel'. We take in four kinds of fuel:

- ♦ food

- ♦ liquid

- ♦ air

- ♦ energy

Macrobiotics also tells us to match our input of each type of fuel with our utilisation of it, so that no unwanted excess builds up within the system. Since our body is a self-regulating, self-balancing system, we can assist it in its task by choosing appropriate fuel for our constitu-tional type and our level of daily activity. This is why there is no single diet, exercise regime or spiritual practice that is suitable for everyone. We are all aware of the adage that 'we are what we eat'. However, what we 'eat' is not simply limited to food but also includes liquid, air and Ki energy.

FOOD

High on the list of requirements for our survival is obviously our intake of food. From a macrobiotic perspective, we should reflect on our own evolution as human beings and try to match the development of this evolution with what we eat. This means basing our daily diet on the use of whole, cooked cereal grains. Wherever you look at traditional diets throughout the world, you will find this central theme. Along with grains, the use of pulses/beans is also common. These provide a source of nutrition in stews or soups and are often combined with whole cereal grains. Local and seasonal vegetables, together with fresh fruit, are also common staples throughout the world. Depending on the climate, some cultures have integrated the use of animal food which could be either game or domesticated animals, and their by-products (cheese/yoghurt), or fish.

The main shift in modern times has been away from whole cereal grains, replacing them with the tuber (potato), and increasing the amount of refined carbohydrates – in the form of sugar and refined (white) flour.

Modern science would argue that food is simply a mass

of chemicals which the body can discern and digest, regardless of its source. Without a doubt, human beings are enormously adaptable regarding diet and, rather like rats, can technically eat anything and survive! However, from a holistic perspective, it is not simply the biochemical source of food that matters but the quality of energy that it provides. Fresh, home-made food, prepared with love, is far more satisfying, sensorily, emotionally and spiritually, than a frozen meal that has been mass-produced in a factory and microwaved in your home or a restaurant.

As far as the impact of food on our biological survival is concerned, it is possible – in extreme circumstances – to actually live without food for anything from 30 to 90 days.

LIQUID

The physical body is made up of roughly 60 per cent fluid and it is important for our health and the electrolyte balance of our system that we neither become overloaded with fluid nor dehydrated. Too much fluid and we can over-stress our already hard-working kidneys, making us feel tired, heavy and lethargic. Too little fluid in our system and the body then has more waste products to deal with, leaving us feeling irritable and uncomfortable.

Water is the most essential element in our liquid consumption, so the important questions to deal with are the source and quality of our water. In traditional times, water would have been drawn from a nearby spring or well. Nowadays there is less choice and water comes to us from the metropolitan supply which is frequently recycled (up to seven times) with chemicals added to neutralise any toxins. Try to find a good source of spring water (bottled if necessary) and use this for making hot drinks, soups and even for preparing your vegetables.

In terms of our survival, liquid is far more important than food. We can only survive five to seven days before we dehydrate, our kidneys fail and we die.

AIR

As far as our daily intake of food and liquid is concerned, at least we have a choice in the quality of what we consume. However, the story is different when it comes to the air we breathe. As the quality of oxygen declines in our major industrialised cities, and the rainforests are destroyed, we are all being affected.

It is really only in our homes and offices that we have some control over our access to fresh air. We can choose whether to exercise or take a walk for 30 minutes every day, we can choose whether or not to smoke, we can choose whether to have oxygen-providing plants in our home, or whether to sleep with the window open or closed at night.

Fresh air is a really vital fuel for our system and we can gain more from this source when we examine *how* we breathe. If you have the opportunity to practise a martial art and take up meditation or yoga, you will notice that almost 90 per cent of the technique is focused on breathing. Opening up the lungs not only oxygenates the blood and our physical system but also leaves us feeling mentally refreshed. Poor breathing, on the other hand, leaves us feeling tired, depressed and even isolated.

From a survival perspective, oxygen is far more important than food and liquid. In comparison to 30 days without food and five or six days without liquid, you will live only three to four minutes without oxygen.

KI ENERGY

Ki is a Japanese term used to describe the life force which is present in a vibrational form in all phenomena within and around us. The Chinese use the word Chi and in India it is known as Prana. Perhaps the nearest equivalent in English is 'spirit'. An easy way to understand how Ki can manifest itself is when you meet an old friend who you haven't seen for some time. You notice straight away whether they appear older, younger, tireder, happy, sad, distracted or calm. There is something about their vibration, something about their energy. In the same way, when you go to select your vegetables at the supermarket, one of the first things that you are looking for is the quality of Ki. Do the vegetables appear fresh or tired and limp?

Rather like food, liquid and air, we all absorb Ki energy. There are two categories of Ki and the first one affects us all. This could include the season that we live in, the climate, the daily weather, the time of day, or any stresses – such as war or economic deprivation – that affect everyone. It is very hard not to be affected by the weather, the climate or the environment in which you live and it is certainly very hard to change these conditions.

The second category of Ki is received on a more individual level – for example the Ki energy of our home, our office environment, our relationships with our colleagues, our family, our children or our spouse. A warm friendly family gathering can uplift your Ki, whereas a family argument can undoubtedly depress your Ki. Since Ki energy permeates every aspect of our lives, it is important that, when given a choice, we go for the most vital and freshest option. We should therefore keep our homes fresh and bright, our clothes clean and fresh, obviously our food as fresh as possible, and our communication with others positive.

Without Ki, our intrinsic life force, we would only survive a millisecond! The importance of food, liquid and air may now seem to pale into insignificance. However, which of these categories do you have the most control over? It is not easy or even possible to control the Ki of your environment or climate, or to determine the quality of air that is being produced on the planet. This is where food, despite being the least important requisite for our survival, plays a major role. It is in this category of fuel that you have the most control, the most responsibility and the greatest choice. A chocolate bar does not simply unwrap itself, fly out of a confectionery shop and land in your mouth! We can all choose what we eat, how we prepare it and how much we eat.

THE DISCHARGE AND ELIMINATION PROCESS

The secret of good health lies in our capacity to utilise and absorb what we take in, while at the same time eliminating what we do not need. Obviously, part of this

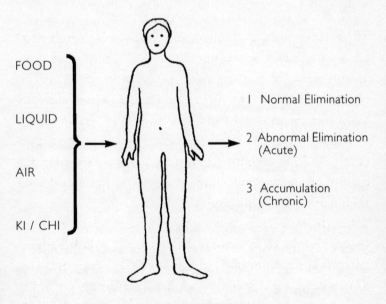

FOOD

LIQUID

1 Normal Elimination

2 Abnormal Elimination (Acute)

AIR

3 Accumulation (Chronic)

KI / CHI

Fuelling the body and the elimination process

process involves selecting the appropriate amount of fuel from the preceding four categories. Proper elimination of toxins and waste from our system helps to prevent the unwanted accumulation of waste which in time can lead to chronic health problems.

Normal Elimination

There are three basic ways in which we all eliminate what we do not need on a daily basis:

♦ through the bowel

♦ through urination

♦ through breathing

These three normal elimination processes are fundamental to us all and the quality and ease of the processes are symptomatic of our general health and well-being. In traditional Chinese medicine, the bowel movement was known as the 'old gold' and the urine was known as the 'new gold'. Even in Western medicine during the eighteenth and nineteenth centuries, it was common for doctors to examine the stools and urine of patients during their ward rounds in hospitals.

Ideally, bowel movements should be regular – once or twice a day, effortless, odourless and gold/brown in colour. Urine should neither be as pale as water nor dark brown but a slight gold colour, like lager beer. Obviously, frequent urination is a sign of too much fluid intake, while small amounts of urine that are very dark and have a strong odour are a sign that you are not drinking enough fluid. As far as breathing is concerned, the obvious signs of health are that you do not get breathless taking simple exercises or going up a flight of stairs, nor do you yawn frequently or have a continuous cough.

Abnormal Elimination

All of us experience abnormal elimination symptoms from time to time. These symptoms may be violent and can be accompanied by a degree of pain or even heat. As we adjust to changing seasons, changes in emotion, or changes in diet or our routine, our system helps to compensate by discharging any excess that is building up. In this situation, our body utilises the same routes as for the normal elimination process (i.e. the bowel, urination and breath) as well as two additional routes that can open up – the skin and our emotions.

It is vital to remember that all these abnormal elimination symptoms are healthy, provided they occur seasonally or as the result of some recent trauma. When they become chronic, however, it means that the body is moving into the third phase (see Chapter 5).

In the Far East these violent elimination processes are regarded as vital to the body's re-balancing process; they help the body rid itself of excess waste and toxins. In the West, however, we may feel encouraged to take some form of medication which will either suppress or neutralise this violent elimination process. While the medication may work effectively to do this, it is simply putting the deeper root cause on hold and undoubtedly the symptoms will recur at a later time, even more violently. In Oriental medicine, when violent elimination occurs, the usual advice is to allow it to run its course and even to encourage it. However, if symptoms of violent elimination persist for 24 hours, accompanied by fever, then this is not elimination but more likely to be an infection and you should consult a doctor immediately.

Symptoms of violent elimination regarding the digestive process include vomiting, diarrhoea, constipation and flatulence. Fluid symptoms include excessive urination and sweating, often accompanied by fever. Violent lung elimination symptoms include coughs, colds, chills and fevers which are not infections. A fourth route can also open up – the skin. In Oriental healing the skin is regarded as either the third lung or the third kidney. Symptoms can include spots, rashes, odour, sweat or fluid. Finally, it is not uncommon, when we are discharging excess waste, to feel uncomfortable emotionally. Short-term expressions of hysteria, complaining, anxiety, depression, fear, irritability or impatience are all common. From an Oriental perspective, it is vital to allow these emotions to be expressed rather than to neutralise and suppress them as they will only be short-lived and do not require in-depth therapy!

Accumulation

In an ideal world, we follow the normal mode of elimination. From time to time, however, as excess waste accumulates, we step into the realm of abnormal or violent elimination to regain balance. For all manner of different reasons, some people find it very difficult to 'let go' and have a tendency to accumulate and store the excess rather than discharging it.

Given time, and given the chronic nature of this inability to discharge, the body will simply take the excess and place it or store it where it can be discharged at a later date. This accumulation can take the form of mucus, fat, cyst, tumour or even calcification in the form of stones. Again, the body is quite remarkable. These accumulations tend to occur firstly where there is space and secondly where there is ultimately an exit from the body. Common sites can include the sinuses, the ears, the lungs, the throat, the stomach, the colon, the small intestine, the liver, the gall bladder, the pancreas, the kidneys, the bladder and the reproductive system.

It is quite common to meet individuals who have practised macrobiotics for between two and five years and who have experienced a major elimination of past accumulated waste. This was not necessarily why they began their practice of macrobiotics. Perhaps it was years and years of the accumulation of fats from cheese or other dairy products that built up within the system and this, over a period of time, in combination with eating macrobiotic quality foods and keeping physically active, caused these old accumulations to discharge. From my own experience, I recall, some nine years after I began my practice of macrobiotics, eliminating a small calcified stone from my sinus! The result was that I could breathe more easily through my nose, began to snore less, and rediscovered a sense of smell that I had not enjoyed since my childhood.

5

THE STAGES OF CHANGE

When you begin your practice of macrobiotics, it is good to be aware of the various stages of change that you go through. From a purely biological perspective, every cell in your body is in a constant state of renewal. As you begin to fuel yourself on a different quality of food, a natural regeneration occurs. And any change, whether social, emotional or biological, is bound to cause upheaval. Understanding the three stages that occur within your blood, whether you are eating macrobiotically or not, will help to explain why you need to be more accurate and disciplined when you begin your practice and can afford to be more liberal later on.

The fundamental change occurs within the blood itself. Broadly speaking, blood can be subdivided into three categories. Firstly, our blood is primarily made up of plasma which accounts for some 50 per cent of its volume. This plasma renews itself every 10 days.

Secondly, some 25 per cent of our blood volume is made up of red blood cells, and, on average, these red blood cells renew themselves every 30 to 40 days. Thirdly, the remaining 25 per cent of our blood is made up of a variety of different white blood cells which can take anything from two to four or even eight months to replace. It therefore takes us all, on average, eight months to completely rebuild and refresh our blood. It is interesting at this point to reflect on what you have been eating these past 10 days or 40 days, or even the past eight months, as it is this food that is currently creating your blood.

STAGE 1: RENEWING THE PLASMA

As with any new project that you may choose to undertake, the initial minutes, hours and days are always the trickiest. In the first 10 days you are replenishing 50 per cent of your blood, so it is important to start with a firm foundation. You therefore need to be very accurate and disciplined at this point. On the other hand, you need to remember that, at this stage in your practice of macrobiotics, you know the least and have the most to learn. It is a frustrating paradox. So, in this first 10 days you should practise with accuracy and not allow yourself to take in any of the old foods that you wish to eliminate from your diet. Eating 90 per cent macrobiotic foods but still taking milk in your tea and having a chocolate bar at 3p.m. daily

39

is enough of a distraction to keep the 'old' blood (plasma) much the same.

Despite all these challenges, it is well worth sticking to your resolution, being clear about your purpose and following any advice or recipes as accurately as possible during these first 10 days. Try to avoid being tempted off the path in this initial phase.

STAGE 2: RED BLOOD CELLS

The initial 10 days can certainly take some adjusting to, as your body craves some of its old fuel and you will probably miss foods that have a familiar texture or taste. After this, the pace of change will begin to slow down. During the second stage, which takes about 30 days, all the red blood cells in your blood will have been rebuilt, based on what you are currently eating.

The first and second stage together take about 40 days. And it is interesting to note how many traditional religions advocate a 40-day period of fasting, prayer, meditation and self-reflection. At the end of the 40-day period, 75 per cent of your blood will have been renewed, giving a new firm biological basis to your health and at the same time allowing a cleansing to occur that goes beyond your blood.

It is during the 30-day second stage that you are most likely to feel the effects of abnormal or violent discharge. It is quite common to experience headaches, fever, digestive upsets, cravings, night sweats, times of depression and despondency, irritability, and potential lethargy (as your body requires more sleep while it undertakes deep internal change).

Many people abandon their practice of macrobiotics during this 30–40 days. If only they had a little more faith in the process and allowed the discharge process to occur, they could then benefit enormously from the deeper work that is going on. During this phase it is really vital to have faith in what you are trying to achieve and to be patient as you work through the somewhat challenging physical and emotional ups and down that everyone experiences.

STAGE 3: WHITE BLOOD CELLS

During this third phase of change, you can relax a bit more and put yourself on 'cruise control'. By now you will have mastered the basics of macrobiotics and been through the more turbulent stages of violent or abnormal discharge. The more physically active you are during Stage 2, the quicker the elimination will occur and the quicker you will work your way through it.

In Stage 3 the changes occur far more slowly. Some 75 per cent of your blood is now built on the new macrobiotic foods and you can afford to relax a little more, can start to incorporate more variety in your cooking, perhaps using some spice or tomatoes or the occasional potato if you wish. It is vital though, even at this stage, to remember that your blood is not yet fully built on macro-biotic foods. Therefore you should not fall back on extremely Yin or extremely Yang quality foods, such as sugar, dairy foods or meats, at this stage. It would be much better to wait eight months, until your blood is 100 per cent built on macrobiotic foods, before trying one of the foods that you used to eat. Then you will truly feel the effect, while at the same time being able to eliminate and discharge it quickly.

IMPROVING YOUR CONSCIOUSNESS

For me, the practice of macrobiotics goes far beyond being choosy about what I eat to sustain my blood. I am also concerned about where and how the foods I eat are produced, how they are prepared, and the quality of blood that I wish to create. For me, the benefits offered by macrobiotics are not only physical stamina, and physical and emotional flexibility and stability, but also clarity, vision and belief in what I say and what I do. There is an undoubted link between our food and our consciousness.

It is easy to see the very real connection, which we all have, with the world around us and how we experience it. Our food is drawn from our environment; our food is in turn transformed into our blood, which then strengthens and replenishes our internal organs. It is only after our blood has been transformed (during the previous three stages which occur over an eight-month period) that it is

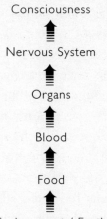

Consciousness

↑

Nervous System

↑

Organs

↑

Blood

↑

Food

↑

Environment / Earth

The link between food and our consciousness

possible for it to get to work on regenerating our internal organs. Deeper, organic change of this nature can take anything from eight months to two years to occur.

Changes can include improved lung and heart function, kidney and liver function, digestive function and the creation of a stronger lymphatic system, reproductive system and immune system. All these changes also filter down to our nervous system. On a practical level, this system allows us to react to change around us, respond quickly and efficiently to new demands and tasks, and look beyond immediate pressures to the new possibilities that lie ahead.

At this stage a whole new side of our being is activated. We can call this level our consciousness, our will, or (as Ohsawa described it) our judgement. In his early works,

George Ohsawa was very preoccupied with what he called the development of our judgement. He rarely wrote about health or cooking or food; these concerns appear far more in his later writing.

Ultimately the true purpose of macrobiotics is to raise our awareness of ourselves, beginning with our individual cells, and then our blood, and culminating with an understanding and appreciation of the world around us. This is why many of the early authors and practitioners of macrobiotics looked far beyond the health of the individual and focused on the wider implications of world health as being fundamental to the realisation of true world peace.

6

ASSESSING YOUR OWN HEALTH STATUS

Your current health is constantly in a state of flux as you adapt to circumstances – your surroundings, your level of activity, your daily diet and the vagaries of the climate. To practise macrobiotics successfully, you need to adapt your diet and lifestyle to maintain a reasonable balance.

In fact, our bodies are quite remarkable natural self-balancing units. Without much effort on our part, they continually work at finding the right electrolyte balance (the appropriate mixture of acid and alkaline) in our blood. But we need to help our bodies, by providing the right fuel, so that they do not waste unnecessary energy and time trying to digest foods that are very demanding and taxing on our systems.

Since your condition is constantly changing, any conclusions you draw from the self-assessment techniques below are only valid at the current time. However, you can use them repeatedly to review your condition at turning points in the calendar (e.g. the Spring and Autumn equinoxes) or when you feel run down. These methods are drawn primarily from Oriental diagnosis and use obvious Yin and Yang examples.

As you go through the list, simply tick off any of the symptoms that seem appropriate to you right now. Naturally, many of the examples are somewhat extreme, and if you do not identify with any of them you can simply ignore them. It is also important to remember that you see the world through your own current condition. This immediately makes any self-assessment exercise a challenge. For instance, what you may consider impatience (relative to your own nature) may not seem so to someone else. It is therefore important to try to be as objective as possible when reviewing your current condition.

You will be able to use the results of this exercise when you look at Chapters 7 and 8 (on the macrobiotic diet and macrobiotic recipes). If, for example, you discover that your current condition is more Yin, then you need to use more ingredients and cooking styles of the opposite nature – Yang – for the first few weeks of your macrobiotic practice. However, it's never advisable to be too extreme and only eat Yang foods or only engage in Yangising activities. The aim is always to create a healthy balance.

SELF-ASSESSMENT TECHNIQUES

Here are eight practical self-assessment techniques that you can use to evaluate your current condition. Remember: only tick the symptom if it is really relevant to you today.

Hands

To establish whether the palms of your hands are moist or dry, pass the back of one hand over the palm of the other one.

- Is the palm of your hand moist? (Yin) ☐
- Is the palm of your hand dry? (Yang) ☐

Fingertips

The extremities of our bodies (Yin) represent and reflect the deeper (more Yang) areas of our body. This exercise can reveal our current internal Yin/Yang condition.

- Are your fingertips bulbous, pink or damp? (Yin) ☐
- Are your fingertips dry, pale or withered in appearance? (Yang) ☐

Feet

The energy that flows through six of the acupuncture meridians begins and ends on our toes and in the soles of our feet. The region around our feet, ankles and toes therefore gives a good indication of Yin or Yang stagnation.

- ♦ Do you have a tendency towards puffy ankles? (Yin) ☐
- ♦ Is your Achilles tendon red/purple or tender? (Yin) ☐
- ♦ Do you have a build-up of hard skin around your heel? (Yang) ☐
- ♦ Are your toenails thick and hard? (Yang) ☐

Cravings

Frequently, as our condition becomes more Yin or Yang, we begin to crave matching foods and tastes. The more Yin our current condition, the more we are then attracted to Yin tastes, flavours, cooking styles and activities. However, once our condition has become a little more balanced, our body is able to send clearer signals as to what we may need to eat or drink at any given time.

- ♦ Are you currently craving coffee, desserts, creamy foods, cold or spicy foods? (Yin) ☐
- ♦ Are you currently craving foods that are dry, savoury, well-cooked or pickled? (Yang) ☐

Sleep Patterns

To get a fair and objective view of your current sleeping pattern, reflect back over the past 10 days and see if you notice any pattern at present. Ignore the occasional

recent night when you may have either slept longer or
shorter than usual, as this could simply be a one-off
occurrence that was necessary at the time. Look at the
general pattern instead.

- Do you have a tendency to sleep for a long period
  at present (7.5 hours plus)? (Yin) □
- Do you generally get up late? (Yin) □
- Do you stay up late and go to bed after midnight?
  (Yin) □
- Do you sleep only for short periods (5–7 hours)?
  (Yang) □
- Do you have difficulty sleeping? (Yang) □
- Do you find yourself waking up before dawn?
  (Yang) □

Urine and Bowel Movements

These two methods of elimination have traditionally
provided, not only in Chinese medicine but also in
Western medicine, vital clues as to our current condition.

- Are you urinating frequently? (Yin) □
- Is the colour of your urine pale? (Yin) □
- Do you urinate infrequently? (Yang) □
- Is the colour of your urine dark or odorous? (Yang) □

- ◆ Do you have frequent bowel movements that are loose and with a strong odour? (Yin) ☐
- ◆ Do you have infrequent bowel movements that are small, hard and dark? (Yang) ☐

Emotions

The way we relate to the outside world and our relationship with others also reflects our current condition. If we are feeling active, lively and impetuous (Yang), then the whole world seems to be too slow. If, on the other hand, we are feeling defensive, tired and vulnerable (Yin), then the outside world will naturally seem threatening.

- ◆ Are you currently feeling worried, fearful or depressed? (Yin) ☐
- ◆ Are you currently feeling irritable, angry or impatient? (Yang) ☐

Symptoms

Finally, run through the following list of symptoms and see if you can identify with any of them. Again, as with the other self-assessment methods, your answers must relate to how you are feeling or expressing yourself *at present*.

- ◆ Are you currently tending to be forgetful, defensive or feeling like a victim? (Yin) ☐
- ◆ Are you currently tending to be rigid, stubborn or forceful in your ideas or opinions? (Yang) ☐

- Are you currently tired? (Yin) ☐
- Are you currently hyperactive? (Yang) ☐
- Are you constantly finding that you are late for appointments? (Yin) ☐
- Do you easily catch cold? (Yin) ☐
- Do you have difficulty sleeping (insomnia)? (Yang) ☐
- Are you finding it difficult in general to relax? (Yang) ☐

CONCLUSION

Having decided whether your current condition is more Yin or Yang, you can begin to adapt the macrobiotic diet (Chapter 7), the lifestyle suggestions (Chapter 9) and the recipes (Chapter 8) to balance your condition.

If you have discovered that your current condition is an even balance of Yin and Yang, then this final additional exercise may help you decide which predominates. This is drawn from the traditional art of Chinese tongue diagnosis. A healthy normal tongue is pink, slightly moist and has a very light coating.

- Is your tongue yellow or red or dry? (Yang) ☐
- Is your tongue pale or white or very wet? (Yin) ☐

7

THE MACROBIOTIC DIET

The Standard Macrobiotic Diet was devised and presented by Michio and Aveline Kushi in the 1970s. This is widely regarded as the benchmark of macrobiotic practice and can be adjusted in terms of proportions, ingredients and cooking styles to suit an individual's condition, the climate they live in, their health or their level of physical activity. The Standard Macrobiotic Diet is also designed for people who live in a temperate 'four seasons climate'. It can naturally be made more Yin (to suit those who live in a hotter, drier climate) or more Yang (to suit those who live in colder, drier or more mountainous regions).

Those ingredients labelled 'Frequent' can be used on a daily basis. Those labelled 'Infrequent' can be used anything from two or three times a week to once or twice a month. 'Infrequent' can also suggest optional. However, it is wise to have as much variety as possible.

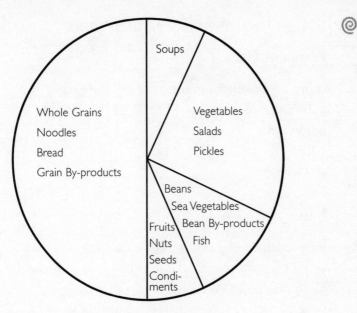

The Standard Macrobiotic Diet

INGREDIENTS

The Glossary at the back of the book explains any unfamiliar terms or ingredients. Some items may be available from healthfood shops, though they tend to specialise more in vitamins and supplements.

Japanese shops may also stock some of the ingredients but it is important to remember that the quality is generally poor compared to what you can find in a natural food shop. The Japanese shops tend to stock only the more refined products and have not, as yet, caught on to the notion of quality organic foods.

Whole Cereal Grains

Frequent Use

short- and medium-grain
  brown rice
pot barley
millet
maize corn

whole oats
wheat berries
buckwheat
rye

Infrequent Use

long-grain brown rice
sweet brown rice
hatto mugi (similar to
  pearl barley)
mochi (pounded sweet
  rice)
bulghur (cracked wheat)
porridge oats
polenta
ryeflakes
couscous

wild rice
quinoa (pronounced
  'keen-wa')
wholewheat noodles
udon noodles
soba noodles (buckwheat)
sourdough bread
pitta bread
fu (wheat gluten)
seitan (wheat gluten)

The basis of the Standard Macrobiotic Diet is the use of whole cooked cereal grains. These have been the traditional staple food of all cultures ever since man discovered fire, began cooking and began to practise agriculture. The traditional grains of northern Europe were oats and rye, which were later supplemented by wheat and barley as the

Celtic influence was felt in the northern regions of Europe. In addition, buckwheat has been used in Russia. Throughout the Middle East wheat and barley have been the staples; in Africa maize corn and millet. In Central and South America quinoa and maize corn are the traditional grains; in India rice and wheat; in China wheat, millet and rice; while in Japan rice has remained the staple.

All the grains listed under 'Frequent Use' are still in their whole form and can be stored for many, many years while retaining their essence. (For instance, some years ago, archaeologists discovered a storage jar of barley buried alongside a mummy in Egypt. They carbon-dated the barley to roughly 3,000 years old and actually succeeded in sprouting some of the grains.) Almost every major culture and religion in the world has a deep appreciation of the use of grain and its by-products. Part of the 'mission' of macrobiotics is to get us to return to the use of this powerful food in our daily life.

To get the most from these whole cereal grains, it is vital that they are cooked. Eating them raw or refined and processed (in the form of flakes, muesli and pasta) takes away their deeper essence. Although this is fine for infrequent use, whole cooked cereal grains need to make up the greater proportion of our intake of grain. Since the dawn of the industrialised era, the use of grain has declined, grains have been further refined, and increasingly they have been used as fodder for livestock – hence the 'meat and two veg' meals which have become so common in the West.

Soups

Frequent Use

miso soup
shoyu broth

Infrequent Use

bean and vegetable soup
brown rice and vegetable
  soup
barley and vegetable soup

millet and vegetable soup
pumpkin soup
noodle and vegetable soup

The Standard Macrobiotic Diet (like the traditional Japanese diet) recommends the daily use of miso soup (see page 87). The basic stock of this soup is made up of the sea vegetable wakame, together with either sautéed or boiled onions and seasonal root or leafy green vegetables. This basic stock is then seasoned with the soya bean fermented purée known as miso. During the lengthy fermentation process, enzymes that aid and settle digestion are formed and this soup – which is frequently eaten for breakfast in Japan – not only helps strengthen the digestive system but also supports the immune system. Small cubes of lightly cooked tofu can also be added and the soup is usually garnished with spring onions, chives or parsley. It is vital to remember not to boil the stock too long once the miso has been added (no more than 2–3 minutes), as this can destroy many of the vital enzymes.

Shoyu Broth (see page 88) can be made by creating a

stock from the sea vegetable kombu, together with dried and pre-soaked shiitake mushrooms and root vegetables. This stock can then be seasoned with naturally fermented soya sauce (shoyu) and garnished with spring onions, chives, parsley or even slices of lemon.

On the 'Infrequent Use' list are many combinations of soups which base their ingredients around vegetables, grains or beans. It is recommended that these are seasoned with good-quality sea salt, shoyu or miso.

The most frequently used miso in macrobiotics is made from barley (mugi) and occasionally miso made from brown rice (genmai) can be used. The very salty pure soya bean miso (hatcho miso) is used less frequently.

Vegetables

Frequent Use

bok choy	daikon greens	radish
(Chinese greens)	daikon root*	red cabbage
broccoli	kale	swede
Brussels sprouts	leeks	spring onions
burdock	lotus root	spring greens
cabbage	(dried or fresh)	turnip
carrots	onion	turnip greens
carrot tops	parsley	watercress
cauliflower	parsnip	
Chinese cabbage	pumpkin	

*This is widely available in the UK in Asian shops and is known as mooli.

Infrequent Use

celery	green beans	shiitake mushrooms
chives	green peas	mangetout
cucumber	lettuce	bean sprouts
dandelion leaves	mushrooms	Jerusalem artichokes

Vegetables can be divided into three categories:

♦ leafy green vegetables

♦ round-shaped vegetables and those that grow at ground level

♦ root vegetables

Try to use all three types in your cooking. Furthermore, try to include a wide variety of vegetables in your daily diet, preparing at least two different vegetable dishes at each meal. One of the dishes could be a pressed salad (see page 127) or a boiled salad (see page 129).

Find a good, preferably organic, source for your vegetables. Never freeze them, as this destroys their vitality. Avoid reheating any previously cooked vegetable dish and always clean the skin of any root vegetable by scrubbing rather than peeling it. The skin and root of root vegetables contain many of the Yang elements (minerals) and it is vital to keep the vegetables 'whole' in order to get the greatest nutrient value from them. Always use a very small amount of sea salt in the cooking to bring out the sweetness, and try different combinations and cooking styles for your vegetables (see pages 127–32).

Beans and Bean Products

Frequent Use

aduki beans	black-eyed beans	pinto beans
black soya beans	kidney beans	soya beans
chickpeas	lima beans	split peas
(garbanzo beans)	mung beans	
lentils (green)		

Infrequent Use

fresh tofu
dried tofu
tempeh
natto

Beans, bean products and fish are the major sources of protein in the Standard Macrobiotic Diet. Traditionally, the combination of cereal grains and beans can be found throughout the world. In many Third World countries, there are dishes that combine corn and beans, rice and beans, rice and peas, rice and lentils, barley stew, hummus and bread, and so on. Research suggests that the humble pea may be the oldest known food crop on the planet – evidence of pea cultivation has been uncovered in Iraq dating back some 5,000 years.

Beans are bought in a dried form. They need to be washed to get rid of any dust and then soaked at room temperature for a period of two to six hours, depending on the bean and the temperature of the water. Beans also need to be cooked for a long time until they are soft enough to be digested easily.

To make beans digestible, they can be boiled together with a small strip of kombu seaweed and a cup of diced root vegetables. This combination can be brought to the boil, and left to simmer for an hour or more, in a heavy stainless steel or cast iron pot. The mixture should only be seasoned with sea salt or shoyu towards the end of the cooking. The best way to test whether your beans are ready to eat is to place one on the tip of your tongue (once it is cool enough!) and see if you can crush it against the roof of your mouth. If you cannot or the bean is still chewy, they are not ready and need further cooking.

Beans can easily be reheated, turned into pâté, or form the basis of a stew or soup the following day. They need to be stored in the refrigerator.

Tofu has been widely used in Japan and China for centuries and is a curd made from soya beans. It is never eaten raw but lends itself well to stir-fries or as an ingredient in stews, and is delicious deep-fried or pan-fried.

Tempeh is a fermented cooked soya bean product that originated in Indonesia. Never eaten raw, it is delicious pan-fried, deep-fried or used as the basis for a stew.

Natto is a fermented soya bean product from Japan that is sticky and has an extremely strong odour. All macrobiotic people are passionate about natto. They either absolutely love it or absolutely detest it! I think it is delicious in salads or combined with a few drops of soy sauce and mustard. It is available (frozen) from Japanese supermarkets.

Sea Vegetables

Frequent Use

wakame
kombu
nori

Infrequent Use

arame
hiziki
dulse
agar agar
Irish moss

Kombu and wakame provide the culinary backbone of most macrobiotically prepared soups and stews. All sea vegetables are high in mineral content and are used in similar ways to animal offal, animal bone or fish, as the basis of soups, stews and stocks. The presence of a small amount of kombu in the preparation of bean dishes helps make them more digestible. Sheets of toasted nori can be used to form the outer layer of a rice ball or sushi, or they can be cut into small slivers and used to garnish soups, stews and grain dishes. Sea vegetables are available from natural food shops.

My initial reaction to the use of sea vegetables was probably like that of most people – revulsion! However, as the basis of a soup or stew, wakame and kombu simply blend into the background. Side dishes made with arame, hiziki, dulse or Irish moss do have a stronger flavour but this is often modified by the combination of the use of seasoning and other vegetables in the recipe.

Agar agar is used like gelatine – to help set both cold summer savoury dishes and sweet fruit jellies (known as kanten).

Fish

Frequent Use

cod	sole	red snapper
haddock	flounder	herring
plaice	trout	whitebait

Infrequent Use

salmon	mussels	shrimps
mackerel	oysters	crab
sardines	prawns	lobster
sprats		

Many individuals choose to practise a vegan version of the Standard Macrobiotic Diet and therefore use no fish whatsoever. Certainly for the first two years that I practised macrobiotics I took no interest in fish; it was only when I began to crave fish that I started to incorporate it.

Living in the UK, the colder, cloudier part of Europe, it is natural to be drawn towards the use of fish. The Scandinavians, Belgians and Dutch, who have a similar climate, also make great use of the oily varieties of fish found in these waters – herring, mackerel and sprats. I personally recommend the use of these oily, small-boned fish in the darker, cooler areas of Europe, as they provide an excellent source of calcium, vitamin D and vitamin B and the essential Omega oils. (During medieval times in Britain, the poor were allowed access to the 'dole', which was the state handout of fresh herring.)

Fish can be steamed, boiled, grilled, baked or even eaten in the Japanese style, raw (as sashimi). To aid the digestion of fish, you should always use an appropriate condiment such as lemon juice, grated daikon or good-quality brown rice vinegar. The Japanese dip their raw fish into a combination of shoyu and wasabi (a form of horseradish that grows close to fresh water) and this combination helps eliminate any parasites that may be lurking in the raw fish flesh.

Pickles

Frequent Use

brine pickles
sauerkraut
pressed pickles

⊚ Infrequent Use

miso pickles
taquan
umeboshi plum

Salty fermented vegetable products are commonly used as an aid to digestion in many traditional cultures. This is especially true where the diet is high in saturated animal fats (e.g. smoked or dried meat, fish or cheese). For example, in Scandinavia and Central Europe there are always pickled vegetables at the table. In the Mediterranean, they may use olives or pickled peppers.

From a macrobiotic perspective, pickles should not be used as an appetiser but as part of the main course, prior to a drink or a dessert. To make life easy, when you begin macrobiotics, I recommend that you find a good source of sauerkraut that simply lists 'cabbage and salt' as the ingredients on the label. Ideally the sauerkraut should be fresh and crunchy. You will need to wash away the excess salt immediately before eating it and you can have anything up to a tablespoon of sauerkraut with your meal.

Taquan is a very salty pickle made from daikan root fermented in miso. I would only recommend one or two very fine slivers of this pickle, perhaps two or three times a week (it is extremely good for the small and large intestine).

Umeboshi plums (which are actually unripe immature

apricots, initially sun-dried and later pickled) taste extremely sour and salty. A quarter of one of these plums, two or three times a week, towards the end of the meal, should suffice.

Try to build up a variety of pickles, always store them in the fridge, and wash them well just prior to eating to remove any excess salt.

Seeds and Nuts

Frequent Use

pumpkin seeds
sesame seeds
sunflower seeds
almonds
peanuts

Infrequent Use

walnuts
hazelnuts

Nuts and seeds can provide a valuable source of oils and fat in the Standard Macrobiotic Diet and, in the case of sesame seeds, calcium. Seeds and nuts should never be eaten raw but lightly dry-roasted in a cast iron pan, which makes them easier to digest, with a few drops of diluted shoyu if you prefer a more savoury snack. Seeds and nuts can be used as a garnish on desserts or to add to a salad, or as the basis (in the case of sesame seeds) of the most traditional of all macrobiotic condiments – Gomashio (see page 149)

As a rough guide, I would recommend no more than ½ cup of toasted nuts per week and no more than 1–1½ cups of toasted seeds per week.

Tahini, nut or seed butters are available from natural food shops.

Fruits

Frequent Use

apples	pears	raspberries
apricots	raisins	strawberries
cherries	plums	blackberries

Infrequent Use

canteloupe melon	watermelon	tangerine
grapes	peach	lemon

Local seasonal fruit is recommended for occasional use (two or three times a week). The fruits can either be eaten raw, or stewed or reconstituted from dried varieties. The juicier fruit (such as watermelons and peaches), and the more tropical in origin (such as tangerines), are regarded as the most Yin. Since all fruit is categorised as being more Yin, it is generally advisable to stick with the more

Yang varieties, such as apples and pears, which are harder and store well for many months.

Traditionally, in temperate climates, fruit was only used seasonally and then it was preserved, either in a dried form or as a jam, for the winter months ahead. Yet it is curious to note that in the tropics the local people do not make fruit the mainstay of their diet – it is frequently used as a snack and often cooked (deep-fried bananas) or even taken with a pinch of salt (as in the case of mango or pineapple).

There is a real myth about the importance of fruit in terms of vitamin C, as we all know that any excess vitamin C we take in is not stored but simply eliminated by the body. In fact, the minimum an adult human being needs is the equivalent daily amount of vitamin C that can be found in one sprig of parsley. This eliminates the need for vast amounts of fruit which can Yinise (or make more acidic) our condition.

In the British diet, for example, we tend to use fruit as a condiment with a heavier, more Yang meat meal. For example, we combine gammon and pineapple, pork and apple sauce, turkey with cranberry, duck with orange, lamb with redcurrant jelly. Traditionally, even the tomato is regarded as a fruit and would be an adjunct to a meal with either steak or, in more recent times, with bacon.

Desserts

Frequent Use

amasake
fruits
kanten (sweet fruit jellies)
kudzu-based desserts

Infrequent Use

cakes*
pies*
crumbles*
* but only sugar- and dairy-free versions from a natural food shop.

This is a challenging area for the would-be practitioner of macrobiotics. If, like me, you were raised on desserts like ice cream, trifles, gateaux and mousse, then you are in for a bit of a sensory surprise! However, there are some very effective desserts that can be made without recourse to chocolate, sugar, dairy products or artificial flavours and colourings. One approach to macrobiotic desserts is to make them appear 'like something that we are sensorily and sentimentally attached to from our previous way of eating'. In my opinion, these desserts are usually a total flop! The ideas I list here (and on pages 138–145) are born out of the Japanese tradition and, with practice, they can be absolutely delicious.

Amasake is made from the fermentation of sweet brown rice, aided by a 'starter' known as koji. It is a similar process to that of making saki (Japanese rice wine) but stops short of actually becoming alcoholic. It can be bought in many natural food shops and resembles creamy rice pudding in appearance. It can be eaten straight from the jar, gently heated up with a few drops of raw ginger oil, or diluted 50/50 with water, heated (again with a few drops of ginger juice) and used as either a custard or a hot drink. As a drink, it can be very relaxing, especially last thing in the evening.

Local seasonal fruits, including dried ones, can be cooked together to form a compote or the basis of a pie or a crumble. When you first start to practise macrobiotics, it is wise to avoid combining oil and flour until your digestive system is stronger. However, if you combine cooked fruits with the Yang Japanese cooking thickening agent known as kudzu, the compote sets and forms a glazed appearance, to which you can add a garnish of chopped nuts or roasted seeds.

Another possibility is to stew fruits gently in apple or pear juice and add agar agar which acts as a form of gelatine. As the mixture cools it will set to form a delicious fruit jelly. If you really enjoy a good mousse, then try putting this cooled product into a blender – the result is deliciously light and fluffy.

Snacks

In your early practice of macrobiotics you may find, like many people, that you are constantly 'peckish'! One of the reasons is that this type and quality of food is very easy to assimilate and you soon start to feel empty. This is by no means unhealthy – it simply takes time to get used to. Secondly, the traditional Western diet (largely based on animal food and potatoes) leaves a sensation of fullness that can last for hours and hours. While the sensation of fullness may be satisfying to some, it can also leave us feeling tired and unenthusiastic. These ideas for macrobiotic snacks can therefore help bridge the gap between meals and can be eaten in the office, at home or while travelling.

Ricecakes, preferably the unsalted ones, can be used as the basis of any snack, any time – either taken plain or dipped into Hummus (see page 109) or a bean pâté or a vegetable dip (see page 135) or a sugar-free jam. Handfuls of nuts and seeds, together with a few well-washed raisins, are also fine. Good-quality wholemeal pitta bread with Hummus (see page 109) or another spread is also fine. Home-made popcorn, either plain or slightly salted, or with fairly liberal amounts of warm barley malt poured over the top and allowed to set, can also make a delicious snack.

My favourite snack, which is quick and easy to prepare, not too heavy so as to spoil a meal and can even be consumed fairly late at night, is buckwheat noodles (soba) with broth. Simply keep a bowl of cooked cold Soba Noodles (see page 103) in the fridge and a jug of Shoyu Broth (see page 88) also in the fridge. It doesn't take a moment to heat up (but not boil) the broth, pour it over a bowl of cold noodles and garnish with spring onions, nori flakes or parsley.

Oils

Frequent Use

sesame oil
toasted sesame oil
corn oil
sunflower oil

Infrequent Use

safflower oil
mustard seed oil
olive oil

Oil is generally used in moderation within the Standard Macrobiotic Diet and cold-pressed oils are always the ones recommended. Traditionally, the Japanese have never been big consumers of oil – simply brushing the pan was enough. However, nowadays they are world-famous for their tempura and this technique of boiling vegetables or fish in oil was actually taught to them by the Portuguese.

Raw oil as a dressing is rarely or never used within the Standard Macrobiotic Diet. A light brushing of a wok or heavy skillet with sesame or dark-roasted sesame oil is enough for most stir-fries or sauté dishes. The use of richer tempura dishes is generally only recommended two or three times a week.

Over the years that I counselled individuals when they began practising macrobiotics, I noticed that after six weeks their main craving was frequently for something 'oily'. When I enquired whether they had had some tempura or stir-fry or sautéed their food regularly, they said they had not. Naturally, after a few weeks, their bodies were craving oil and they soon found themselves standing on the threshold of their local fish and chip shop literally drooling! By simply being inventive, creative and taking the time to use oil in moderation in your diet, you can naturally lessen your desire to go for the more extreme uses of oil.

Drinks

Frequent Use

bancha twig tea (kuki cha)	spring water
roasted barley tea	cereal grain coffee
roasted brown rice tea	

Infrequent Use

mu tea	soya milk
carrot juice	beer (Guinness or natural
apple juice	ale)
bancha leaf tea	warm saké
(green tea)	white wine
dandelion coffee	whisky

The most common beverage within the Standard Macrobiotic Diet is Bancha Twig Tea (see page 148). This is a refreshing drink which can be heated and re-used time and time again.

There are many grain-based coffee substitutes in most natural food shops but I would advise against using coffee that has been decaffeinated. Do find a source of good-quality spring water to use, not only as a drink but for the basis of your hot drinks and soups. Certainly don't over-indulge in fruit juices – they are best consumed at room temperature or even warmed up. Macrobiotic people are certainly not averse to the odd alcoholic drink but again these are best taken at room temperature and in modera-tion. Soya milk is extremely Yin and therefore has a very cooling effect on our bodies. It is best taken warm or you can put a few drops into a hot drink if you are missing a creamy flavour. If you are very susceptible to the effects of caffeine don't have too much bancha leaf tea (green tea), as it is quite high in caffeine.

The most important point is to drink a comfortable amount of liquid every day to quench your thirst. As you adjust to this way of eating, your desire for liquid may increase or decrease, depending upon your condition. There is no set amount of liquid that you should consume on a daily basis.

Seasonings

Frequent Use

unrefined white sea salt
shoyu
barley miso (mugi miso)
pure soya bean miso (hatcho miso)

Infrequent Use

lemon juice	ginger juice
tamari	umeboshi plum or paste
brown rice vinegar	umeboshi vinegar
mirin	garlic

Access to good-quality unrefined white sea salt is essential in your practice of macrobiotics. Ask in your local natural food store for the best quality – I prefer to use the finer rather than the coarser version.

As far as miso is concerned, look for organic and unpasteurised varieties that have been fermented for at least 24 months.

Regarding shoyu, read the label carefully and look for

a variety that has been fermented for at least 18 months. Never use any of these very Yang products raw at the table.

A frequent criticism of macrobiotics is that it is too heavy in salt. This is really not the case, provided you follow the recipes carefully and remember never to add any of these products raw to your cooked foods. They should always be used in small amounts, generally towards the end of the cooking process.

Ginger is most frequently used in the form of ginger juice. To make this, take a piece of unpeeled ginger root, grate it and squeeze the juice out of the grated ginger.

Brown rice vinegar or umeboshi vinegar can provide a pleasant dressing for Pressed Salad (see page 127) or Boiled Salad (see page 129), and ginger is delicious in soups and stews. Garlic, as we know, has quite remarkable qualities but, from a Yin/Yang perspective, garlic is also quite extreme. Traditionally, garlic was used in combination with heavier animal fat based dishes to help clean the digestive tract. Taken simply on its own, with a vegetable-quality diet, it may cause some intestinal discomfort. The best way of removing some of the strong Yin elements from the garlic, while maintaining some of the Yang qualities which can be beneficial, is to peel a clove of garlic and bury it in half a teacup of raw miso. Steep it in the miso for at least 10 days in the refrigerator and then use a small amount from time to time in your cooking if you feel that it will give sensory or sentimental support – it reminds you of what you ate as a child or the food that you generally enjoy or are used to – to any of the dishes you are eating.

Condiments

Frequent Use

gomashio (sesame salt)
roasted wakame powder
goma wakame powder
(sesame seeds and wakame)

nori flakes
tekka (a root vegetable and
   miso condiment)
umeboshi plums

Infrequent Use

umeboshi vinegar
brown rice vinegar
shiso powder

nori condiment
shio kombu

One of the most frequently asked questions regarding the Standard Macrobiotic Diet is 'How can I adjust my diet to suit my condition in terms of Yin and Yang?' Obviously, cooking styles, volumes and ingredients, proportions of foods and recipes can all help you make these adjustments but the real secret is the use of condiments. These are a wonderful example of Yin and Yang. Something so small, potentially salty and definitely Yang can adjust the overall picture.

However, if you are changing to macrobiotics from a savoury, salty, Western diet then do not be tempted to add too many condiments to your meals. Try your best to follow the guidelines and wait for your system to adjust to the new regime. (This usually takes 10–30 days.)

The most commonly used condiment is Gomashio (see page 149). This delicious, nutty, savoury condiment can be used on cooked grains, but never more than ½–1 teaspoon per day.

Roasted wakame powder is easy to make: simply dry-roast the wakame in the oven and crush it in a suribachi. To make goma wakame, take the roasted, ground wakame and mix it with 5 parts toasted sesame seeds to 1 part roasted wakame powder.

Nori flakes can be bought in most natural food shops and a small sprinkling of these over cooked grains is delicious and tangy. Tekka is a very strong condiment and I do not recommend more than ⅛–¼ teaspoon two or three times a week on cooked grains.

The more unusual condiments, such as nori, need to be used cautiously – only 1–2 teaspoons with a meal, no more than three or four times a week. Nori also needs to be stored in the refrigerator.

Similarly, with shiso powder, a small sprinkling, say ¼ teaspoon, is plenty; and you should limit yourself to two or three times a week.

Shio kombu are small 2.5cm (1 inch) squares of kombu that have been boiled in soy sauce for at least 40 minutes. One or two of these squares, rinsed in water first, can be taken, perhaps two or three times a week to aid digestion.

Condiments form a vital part of the Standard Macrobiotic Diet but, as I have already said, you should neither over-indulge in them nor completely ignore them. With skill and practice, you can master their use and adjust your diet accordingly.

HEAT SOURCE

When learning about macrobiotic cookery people frequently ask what kind of cooker they should use. Given that nowadays we have a choice of gas, electric or microwave, the ideal macrobiotic heat source is gas. I am especially fond of bottled gas, as the flame is much mellower than metropolitan mains gas which is a lot fiercer and more difficult to control.

The reason for this preference for gas is that (unlike electricity or microwave) it actually has a flame which is not dissimilar to the flame used by our ancestors to prepare food. A good question to ask yourself is 'What does a flame represent?' The answer lies in our evolution as human beings. The major turning point for mankind was our discovery of fire. This gave us the possibility of cooking, which led to us beginning to farm, to communicate and to what we call become 'civilised'.

The flame is simply a microcosm of what nurtures all of us – the sun. There is something intrinsically life-giving about using a flame – which is not the case when you use electricity or a microwave. It's rather like being given a choice between attending a Beethoven concert or listening to it being played live on the radio. Essentially, what hits your eardrum is exactly the same but the soul and the experience of the event is totally different.

As far as the use of microwave is concerned, I regard this as purely an experiment at present. We have had very little experience of living with this cooking style, whereas for thousands of years we have cooked our food from the outside towards the inside. Microwave cookery does exactly the opposite, thus Yinising rather than Yangising in the cooking process. In addition, we are all still unclear about microwave energy and its effect on our food and health.

We know that direct exposure to microwave energy can be dangerous and direct electromagnetic energy, as used in telecommunications and in an oven, can burn. In 1992 the National Radiological Protection Board reviewed evidence of electromagnetic fields and cancer risks. Their view was that more research was needed as they could not conclude that electromagnetic fields had no effect on the physiology of cells or that they did not produce effects that would be regarded as potentially carcinogenic.

However, in a microwave oven we are not exposed to its electromagnetic radiation and they are regarded as safe. But how safe? It is, like mobile phones, too early in our culture to know for sure what the long-term effects may be. The jury is still out. My advice would be to leave microwaves alone.

Apart from your choice of heat source, remember that your kitchen creates not only your food but your blood, your health and vitality. It is therefore important that your kitchen represents your dream of good health. I always suggest that when you begin macrobiotics you have a good spring-clean – clear away all the products that you will no longer be using and start to make it a peaceful environment to work from.

From a Feng Shui perspective, it is always wise to position yourself in the kitchen when you are preparing your food so that you can clearly see the door from where you work. This gives you a sense of calm and reassurance that no one is coming up from behind to surprise you. Equally, you should also position yourself away from 'direct traffic' through the kitchen. Many modern kitchens have a door into the garden and you may find yourself being constantly disturbed and distracted by other members of the household.

It's also best to avoid placing the cooker under a roof light or up against a window area. The Ki from the food can be dissipated, like smoke, up a chimney.

When you do spring-clean your kitchen, pay particular attention to the 'cupboard under the sink'. This often houses a vast array of deadly materials designed to kill ants, flies and wasps and unblock drains using all kinds of dreadful chemicals! Since your kitchen is a haven of peace and a source of your future health, even the humble 'cupboard under the sink' should reflect this.

COOKING UTENSILS

It is a lot easier to learn and begin to prepare macrobiotic foods if you have the right pots, pans and cooking utensils. Ideally, you need a stainless steel pressure cooker, two or three stainless steel pots with heavy bases and tight-fitting lids, a heavy cast iron pan with a lid, a stainless steel wok and at least one heavy cast iron casserole pot. To these basic pots and pans I would add a stainless steel collapsible steamer for reheating rice and steaming vegetables.

Since many macrobiotic dishes require low, quiet cooking styles on a low flame, I would invest in some form of flame diffuser to place between the flame and the base of the pan. Add to this a good-quality stainless steel grater, a vegetable brush for scrubbing the vegetables and a variety of wooden spoons and spatulas to use in your pristine stainless steel pots.

The ultimate tool in a macrobiotic kitchen is a kitchen knife and appropriate sharpener. I personally like to use a Japanese vegetable knife which at first sight may seem large, potentially dangerous and cumbersome. You will soon learn how to use it but make sure you hide it from anybody else in the household who might be tempted to think that it's a useful cleaver!

Two other particularly useful items are a sushi mat and a suribachi. A sushi mat is made from thin strips of bamboo woven together to make a flexible base which can be used to roll sushi. It can also be used to cover food

81

by being placed over the top of a bowl. They are available in Chinese and Japanese shops, good natural food shops and by mail order from Clearspring Direct (see page 185).

A suribachi is a tough, earthenware bowl, usually brown in colour, which has fine ridges on the inside. It comes with a wooden pestle (surikogi) and can be used to gently grind seeds and nuts and purée foods such as miso. They are also available from Clearspring Direct.

STORAGE

I prefer to keep grains, beans, sea vegetables, seeds, nuts, dried fruits, salt, flakes and flours in well-sealed glass jars at room temperature. Shoyu oil, brown rice vinegar and umeboshi vinegar will all keep on the counter at room temperature. However, miso I would keep in the refrigerator, along with fresh salads and vegetables. Soup stocks, bean dishes and stews are also best kept in the fridge, but not cooked brown rice.

Cooked rice has a tendency to dry out and I never recommend storing it in plastic containers in the fridge. The best way to keep and store your cooked brown rice is to transfer it to a wooden fruit or salad bowl that you have previously lightly oiled on the inside with a modest amount of sesame oil. Once the rice is in the bowl, place one umeboshi plum very deep into the centre of the rice and cover the bowl with a slightly damp cotton cloth. Keep the bowl in the coolest part of the kitchen but do

not be tempted to leave it in the refrigerator. Provided the
kitchen is not too hot, rice can be kept in this way for two
or three days.

VARIETY AND FRESHNESS

Variety in cooking, as in any aspect of our lives, is vital for
bringing a sense of spark into whatever we choose to do.
Variety in macrobiotic cooking means: a variety of
cooking styles, a variety of ingredients, a variety of
colours, a variety of tastes, a variety of ingredients, a
variety of condiments, and a variety of volume of food.
Those who rarely eat the same dish twice, who are adven-
turous with their cooking, are the ones who succeed in
the long term in their practice of macrobiotics.

Stale food is like stale air or water – uninspiring. When
we eat freshly prepared food (rather than reheated or
factory packaged foods) we feel alive and alert. The more
Yang components of the macrobiotic diet – soups, stews,
beans and grains and sea vegetables – do allow themselves
by their constitution to be reheated. However, it is
among the Yin ingredients – vegetables, salads and fruits
– that this concept of freshness needs to be applied.
Always find the freshest source of vegetables, salads and
fruits; prepare them as soon as possible; and, whatever is
left, do not be tempted to store and reheat. The light,
fresh Yin energy of these ingredients will be lost through
lengthy preparation time, pressure and reheating.

RESOURCES AND RESEARCH

None of us are likely to have had the privilege of having a macrobiotic mother, aunt or neighbour to show us the ropes. We all tend to learn our cooking from our mothers or grandmothers. So, when you begin to practise macrobiotics, you really need to find a surrogate macrobiotic mother! She may come in the form of a wonderful individual who patiently teaches the art of macrobiotic cookery. Find out if there is a macrobiotic cookery course close to you, sign up, watch, listen, observe and enjoy. It is an art but one not to be over-awed by.

Deep down, we are all capable of mastering our own cooking; and in many ways the less you know about cooking, the better. In this sense you are far more trainable and coachable than someone who already knows how to cook. If you have little or no knowledge of cooking, then you have no bad habits to iron out and can be taught right from the beginning how to prepare food. Likewise, if you do know a lot about cooking, you should attend the class as if you were five years old and know absolutely nothing (to avoid the frustration of trying to integrate your previous knowledge of cooking styles and techniques).

Other good sources of knowledge are the many excellent macrobiotic cookery books and the helpful insights and advice that you can gain at your local natural food shop. Once you have mastered the basics of the cooking, the best research you can undertake (apart from on yourself) is to prepare a meal for a friend, a relative or a neigh-bour.

When you prepare the food with love, and focus in on their particular needs without making a big deal about it, the meal always ends up being a success. Where it can all fall apart is when you begin to lecture your guests about the importance of using brown rice and why they should not be eating any more dairy food or sugar or animal products in their diet. None of us like to feel threatened by other people's ideas and opinions, and close members of your family are bound to be a bit suspicious of your strange new interest in preparing foods that look completely alien to what you were raised on.

The best way to inspire anybody else in your own prac-tice of macrobiotics is through your being. People close to you will notice if you look different, are more flexible, livelier, or have a sparkle in your eye. Their curiosity is going to be far greater if you keep quiet about what you are up to!

8

MACROBIOTIC RECIPES

The following recipes have been carefully prepared by Bob Lloyd, one of the finest macrobiotic cooks I know. His enthusiasm for creating macrobiotic meals really shines out when you attend his cookery classes or dinner parties. We have specially chosen, researched and tested the following recipes for their rich flavour and variety (both important factors when you begin to practise macrobiotics).

There are suggestions for breakfast dishes, soups, main meals and, of course, desserts. A majority of the recipes are 'balanced' in terms of Yin and Yang. However, where indicated, certain dishes definitely lean more towards the Yin and others more towards the Yang and these have been highlighted.

Having established whether your current condition is more Yin or more Yang (see Chapter 6), you can choose your menu accordingly. If, for example, your condition leans more towards Yin, then select any of the recipes that are not highlighted and include a few Yang ones. In addition to this, you could increase your use of condiments by some 50 per cent from the list on page 76.

If your condition is predominantly Yang, then you should use any of the recipes that are not highlighted and emphasise any that are predominantly Yin. Make sure that you only use a moderate amount of the condiments recommended on page 76 and do not be tempted to over-season your food with either shoyu, miso or sea salt.

Enjoy!

Measurements
1 tablespoon = 15ml
1 dessertspoon = 10ml
1 teaspoon = 5ml

SOUPS

All the soup recipes serve 4–6.

Vegetable Miso Soup

This is easy to make – and tastes great too!

a little sesame oil or sunflower oil	1 x 12cm (5in) strip wakame
2 onions, peeled and finely sliced	1–1½ tablespoons miso (preferably
2 carrots, scrubbed and finely diced	mugi miso)
2 sticks celery, finely sliced	2 spring onions, finely sliced

1. Heat the oil in a saucepan and fry the onions until soft but not browned. Add the carrots and celery and stir for 1 minute. Add 1.2 litres (2 pints) cold water, bring to the boil, cover and simmer for 10 minutes.

2. Rinse the wakame and soak in 90–120ml (3–4fl oz) cold water for a few minutes until soft enough to slice finely. Add to the soup, together with the soaking liquid. Simmer for 5 minutes.

3. Place the miso in a bowl and blend with a little soup stock into a smooth purée. Add to the soup and simmer, uncovered, for 2–3 minutes, taking care not to let it boil. Serve garnished with the spring onion.

Shoyu Broth

An ideal soup for winter evenings.

1 x 8cm (3in) strip kombu	2 sticks celery, diagonally sliced into
2 dried shiitake mushrooms	0.5cm (1/4in) strips
1 onion, peeled, halved and sliced	2–3 tablespoons shoyu
1 large carrot, scrubbed and sliced	finely sliced spring onions, chives, celery
into 0.5cm (1/4in) rounds	or lemon to garnish

1. Wipe the kombu with a damp cloth and place in a large pan with 1.2 litres (2 pints) cold water and the shiitake mushrooms. Soak for about 10 minutes. When softened, remove the shiitake, discard the stalks, finely slice the tops and then return them to the pan.

2. Add the vegetables and bring to the boil gently. Simmer for 5 minutes and remove the kombu. (Keep the kombu in the fridge as it can be reused.) Simmer for a further 5 minutes and add the shoyu. Continue to simmer for 2 more minutes and then serve with a garnish of your choice.

VARIATION

This broth can also be served cool in summer, garnished with lemon and parsley.

YIN   *Cauliflower and Lemon Soup*

An unusual, but delicious soup that can be served hot or chilled.

1 medium cauliflower (approx. 500g/	1¹/₂–2 tablespoons white miso
1lb 2oz)	juice of 1 lemon
1–2 onions, peeled and diced	chopped parsley
a pinch of sea salt	

1. Cut the cauliflower into small pieces, using some of the stalks as well – finely sliced.

2. Place the diced onions in a pot and put the cauliflower on top. Add 850ml (1¹/₂ pints) water and a pinch of sea salt and bring to the boil. Simmer until the vegetables are soft – about 20 minutes.

3. Cool a little and blend with a potato masher. Return to the heat and add white miso to taste, plus the lemon juice. Simmer gently for 1 minute. Serve garnished with the parsley.

VARIATIONS

If you do not have white miso, mugi miso or sea salt will be fine, and sauerkraut juice can be substituted for the lemon juice.

Pumpkin Soup

A wonderfully creamy soup that couldn't be simpler to make.

2 medium onions peeled, halved
 and sliced
1 medium pumpkin, peeled and
 cut into small chunks
a pinch of sea salt

a little mirin *or* ginger juice (optional)
1–2 tablespoons white miso *or*
 mugi miso
toasted nori, cut into small squares

1. Place the onions in a pan and cover with the pumpkin chunks. Cover the vegetables with 850ml (1½ pints) water, add a pinch of salt and bring to the boil. Simmer uncovered for 5 minutes, then cover and simmer until the vegetables are very soft (about 20 minutes).
2. Remove the pan from the heat and allow to cool a little, before blending into a purée. Add a little more water if it is too thick. Season to taste with mirin or ginger juice (see page 75) and miso and return to the heat. Simmer gently for 5 minutes. Serve garnished with the nori squares.

VARIATIONS

In summer, you can replace the pumpkin with squash. In winter, try sautéing the onion in a little sesame oil before adding the other ingredients.

Lentil Soup

175g (6oz) green or brown lentils

2 onions, peeled and diced

2 sticks celery, sliced

2 carrots, scrubbed and diced

1 x 12cm (5in) piece wakame

1½ tablespoons miso

a little ginger juice (see page 75)

a few spring onions, finely sliced on the diagonal

1. Pick over, wash and drain the lentils. Prepare the vegetables and place them in a saucepan – onions first, then celery and finally the carrots.
2. Next add the sliced wakame, which should be rinsed and soaked in a little cold water first. Place the lentils on top, plus the soaking water from the wakame and 1.2 litres (2 pints) water. Bring to the boil, reduce the flame, cover and simmer until the lentils are soft (about 45 minutes).
3. Add the miso, puréed in a little of the soup liquid, and continue to simmer very gently for 3–4 minutes. Add the ginger juice and allow to cook for just 1–2 minutes longer.
4. Serve garnished with the spring onion.

French Onion Soup with Garlic Croutons

This is a delicious version of the traditional recipe

2 tablespoons olive oil

6 large onions, peeled, halved and finely sliced

a pinch of sea salt

1 x 12cm (5in) strip of kombu

2–4 tablespoons shoyu

freshly ground black pepper

2 cloves garlic, peeled and minced

2 thick slices wholemeal bread (preferably sourdough), cut into croutons

1 tablespoon chopped parsley

1. Heat 1 tablespoon of the olive oil in a large, heavy pan and add the sliced onions. Sauté for a few minutes and turn the heat very low. Add a pinch of salt and cover the pan. Allow the onions to sweat very gently until they are reduced to a very soft mush. Stir from time to time so that they do not brown. Add a little extra olive oil or a tablespoon of water if they are catching in the pan.

2. Add the kombu and 850ml (1½ pints) cold water to the onions, bring to the boil and simmer, covered, for 15 minutes. Remove the kombu and save for further use. Season with shoyu and black pepper and simmer for 5 minutes.

3. In a frying pan, heat the remaining olive oil and add the garlic and the bread. Fry until crisp and golden, stirring and turning the croutons once or twice. Remove from the pan and drain on kitchen paper.

4. Serve the soup garnished with the croutons and parsley.

Minestrone Soup ◎

A great Italian classic.

1 tablespoon sesame or olive oil	1 tablespoon chopped parsley
1 onion, peeled and diced	freshly ground black pepper
1 stick celery, sliced	mugi miso (optional)
2 carrots, scrubbed and sliced	1 cup (175g/6oz) cooked pasta
a pinch of sea salt	1 cup (175g/6oz) cooked kidney beans

1. Heat the oil in a large pan and add the onion. Sauté for 2 minutes, then add the celery and carrots. Add a pinch of salt and simmer covered, very gently, for 10 minutes, stirring from time to time.
2. Add the parsley and 850ml (1½ pints) cold water. Bring to the boil and simmer, covered, for 20 minutes. Season with salt and pepper, and simmer for 2 minutes. (If using miso, purée 1–2 tablespoons miso with a little of the soup stock and add to the pan. Simmer gently for 2 minutes without boiling.)
3. Add the pasta and kidney beans and gently heat through before serving.

GRAINS, PASTA AND NOODLES

YANG *Pressure-cooked Brown Rice*

SERVES 4

2 cups (375g/13oz) brown rice

3 cups (750ml/1¼ pints) water

2 pinches of sea salt

1. Wash the rice and drain thoroughly. Place in a pressure cooker and gently add the cold water. Slowly bring to a simmer, uncovered. Add the salt and put the lid on the pressure cooker. Bring to pressure and place over a ready-heated flame diffuser. Reduce the heat to very low and cook for 45–50 minutes.

2. Remove from the heat and allow the pressure to come down naturally. Open the pan and transfer the rice to a bowl with a wet rice paddle or wooden spoon, mixing it gently. Cover with a sushi mat or a tea towel until needed.

3. If you do not have a pressure cooker, cook in a heavy, covered pan for 50–60 minutes using 4 cups (850ml/1½ pints) water. Boiling makes the recipe more Yin.

Brown Rice with Chestnuts ◎

Chestnuts are the lowest-fat nuts, making this a very healthy recipe.

SERVES 6

2 cups (375g/13oz) short-grain brown rice
½ cup (75g/3oz) sweet rice (see Glossary)
110g (4oz) dried chestnuts, soaked in 2 cups (450ml/³/₄ pint) cold water for 2
 hours
2 pinches of sea salt

1. Wash both types of rice, drain and place with the chestnuts in a pressure cooker. Add the chestnut soaking water and enough extra water to make up to 3³/₄ cups (850ml/1½ pints). Bring to the boil, add the salt, cover and bring to pressure.
2. Place a flame diffuser under the pot, reduce the flame to a minimum and cook for 45 minutes.
3. Remove from the heat and allow the pressure to come down naturally. Spoon into a bowl, mix gently and serve.

Sushi

For each sushi you will need:

1 sheet toasted (sushi) nori
about 1 cup (175g/6oz) cooked
 short-grain rice
brown rice vinegar

1 strip of carrot and 1 strip of
 cucumber the same length as the nori sheet
tahini and sauerkraut or wasabi (or
 mustard) and umeboshi purée

1. Place the nori, shiny side down, on a sushi mat. Take the rice and, with moistened hands, press it gently and evenly over the nori, leaving a 1–2cm ($\frac{1}{2}$–1in) space at the end furthest from you (top) and a 0.5cm ($\frac{1}{4}$in) space on the end nearest to you (bottom). Sprinkle some brown rice vinegar over the rice.

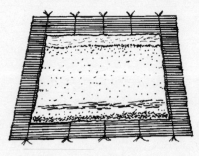 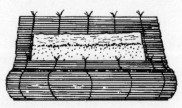

I. Lay nori horizontally on square sushi mat

2. Begin rolling nori with aid of mat

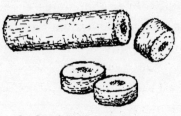

3. Carefully slice into desired thickness

How to assemble sushi

2. Boil the carrot strip for 4–5 minutes, drain and cool, then place this lengthwise about 2.5cm (1in) in from the bottom end of the rice. Place the cucumber strip

next to the carrot and then use your chosen flavourings as follows. For tahini and sauerkraut sushi, spread the tahini along the vegetables with a spoon and then top with some drained sauerkraut. For wasabi and umeboshi sushi, mix the wasabi into a paste with a little cold water. Spread this, and the umeboshi purée, along the vegetables with a teaspoon. You need about 1 level teaspoon of the umeboshi and $\frac{1}{4}$ teaspoon of wasabi for each sushi. (You can replace the wasabi with mustard if you wish.)

3. Start to roll up the sushi from the bottom, making sure that the vegetables stay in place. Exert firm pressure as you continue rolling and remember to pull the end of the sushi mat out as you go along.

4. When completely rolled, moisten the end of the nori and press to seal along its length. Take a very sharp knife and moisten it. Slice the sushi into 6–8 pieces, using a saw-like motion and wetting the knife between each slice. If you use a dry knife, the nori will tear.

5. Serve with Ginger Dip (see below). When travelling, you can cut the sushi roll into just 2 pieces, rewrap it in the mat and place in a paper bag.

Ginger Dip Sauce for Sushi

This is also good with noodles or fried foods like tempura.

1 tablespoon fresh ginger juice (see page 75)
2 tablespoons shoyu or tamari soy sauce
1 tablespoon mirin

1. Put the ginger juice in a bowl and add the other ingredients, as well as 3–4 tablespoons cold water. Stir well and serve as a dip with your sushi rolls.

YIN Rice Salad

SERVES 3–4

1 cup (150g/5oz) broccoli florets
3 large carrots, scrubbed and diced
3 sticks celery, diced
a pinch of sea salt
3 cups (350–450g/12oz–1lb) cooked
  brown rice
1/2 cucumber, quartered and sliced

2 tablespoons finely chopped
  sauerkraut
2–3 tablespoons toasted sesame oil
1–2 tablespoons brown rice vinegar
1/2–1 tablespoon shoyu
1 tablespoon finely chopped parsley

1. Cook the broccoli, carrots and celery in boiling water with a pinch of salt for 1–2 minutes, refresh under cold water and drain well.
2. Fluff up the cooked rice in a bowl and mix in the vegetables, cucumber and sauerkraut. Mix the oil, vinegar and shoyu together and stir into the salad. Garnish with parsley and serve.

YANG   *Millet*

Millet is good for digestion and packed with nutrients.

SERVES 4–6

2 cups (400g/14oz) millet

2 pinches of sea salt

some roasted pumpkin seeds, roughly chopped (optional)

sesame oil (optional)

1. Wash the millet in a sieve and drain thoroughly. Dry-roast it in a frying pan, stirring constantly to avoid burning. When there is a nutty aroma and all the grains have turned golden, add to a pan holding 5–6 cups (1.2–1.5 litres/2–2½ pints) boiling water. Add the salt, cover, reduce heat to very low and simmer for about 30 minutes on a flame diffuser.

2. Remove from the heat, place in a bowl and fluff up with a fork. When cool enough to handle, you can form the millet into patties if you wish. Serve with a garnish of roughly chopped roasted pumpkin seeds or fry the patties in a little hot sesame oil.

VARIATION

You can also cook vegetables with the millet – add some onion, carrot or pumpkin. Or cook with cauliflower florets equal in volume to the dry millet, and mash together after cooking to create a 'mashed potato' effect.

YIN **Bulgur Wheat Salad**

SERVES 4–6

1 small onion, peeled and diced

1 small green pepper, diced

2 carrots, scrubbed and diced

a pinch of sea salt

2 cups (450g/1lb) bulgur wheat

½ cucumber, diced

2 tablespoons shoyu

2 tablespoons rice vinegar or cider vinegar

2 tablespoons toasted sesame oil or olive oil (optional)

1 tablespoon chopped coriander or parsley

1. Bring 3 cups (750ml/1¼ pints) water to the boil in a pan and add the onion, green pepper, carrots and salt. Bring back to the boil and add the bulgur wheat. Cover the pan and turn the heat very low. Simmer until all the liquid has evaporated (about 15–20 minutes).

2. Remove from the heat and place the bulgur and vegetables in a bowl. Add the cucumber, shoyu, vinegar, oil (if using) and chopped coriander or parsley. Mix gently together and serve.

Couscous

Couscous is a traditional grain from North Africa.

SERVES 3–4

1 tablespoon sesame oil

1 onion, peeled and diced

2 cups (375g/13oz) couscous

2 pinches of sea salt

1 tablespoon chopped parsley

1. Heat the oil and sauté the onion in a saucepan. Cook just enough to soften, then take the pan from the heat and add 750ml (1¼ pints) water carefully. Bring to the boil, stir in the couscous and add a pinch of sea salt. Gently return to the boil, remove from the heat and cover tightly. Leave the lid on for 20 minutes.

2. Place the couscous in a bowl, breaking up any lumps. Sprinkle with parsley and serve with your favourite sauce (see pages 136–8) or stew.

Quinoa

This is as close to a perfect food as you can get – high in protein, rich in vitamins and minerals and low in fat.

SERVES 2–3
1 cup (175g/6oz) quinoa, washed and drained
a pinch of sea salt

Note: It is essential to wash quinoa very thoroughly before use, as it can be gritty and may taste bitter otherwise. Place the grain in a large, fine-mesh sieve, hold under a fast-running cold tap and mix about with your fingers to clean. Then leave to drain for a few minutes before cooking.

1. Place the quinoa and salt in a saucepan with 2 cups (500ml/¾ pint) cold water. Cover and bring to a simmer. Turn flame to low and cook for 15 minutes until all the liquid has been absorbed.

2. Place in a bowl, fluff up with a fork and serve with Simple Bean Stews (page 110), salads, sauces (pages 132–8), or use to stuff mushrooms or peppers. Alternatively, try the following recipe.

Quinoa Pilaf

SERVES 4–6

2 tablespoons sesame oil

1 onion, peeled and diced

2 cloves garlic, peeled and minced (optional)

2 carrots, scrubbed and diced

2 cups (350g/12oz) quinoa, washed and drained

¼ teaspoon sea salt

freshly ground black pepper

2 tablespoons shoyu

juice of 1 lemon

1 tablespoon chopped parsley

1. Heat the oil in a heavy pan and add the onion. Sauté gently for about 5 minutes, then add the garlic if using. Sauté for a minute and add the carrots. Continue to sauté for a further 2 minutes, then add the quinoa.
2. Keep stirring for 3–4 minutes, then add 4 cups (1 litre/1¾ pints) hot water, salt and pepper. Bring to a simmer, cover the pan and reduce the flame to very low. Cook until all the liquid has been absorbed (about 15–20 minutes). Turn off the flame and leave the pan untouched for 5 minutes.
3. Now transfer the pilaf to a bowl and fork through gently. Add the shoyu and lemon juice and mix in carefully. Sprinkle with the parsley and serve.

YANG ## *Soba Noodles* ◎

These taste great on their own, or with a sauce (see pages 136–8), dips (see pages 134–5) or in soups and broths (see pages 87–93).

SERVES 4

1 x 200g (7oz) packet 40% soba (buckwheat) noodles

Note: Do not add salt as Japanese noodles are already salted.

1. Add noodles gradually to about 8 cups (2 litres/3½ pints) fast-boiling water and stir gently. Bring back to the boil but keep watching as they can easily boil over. If this starts to happen add some cold water. This is called 'shocking', and if you do this three times the noodles will usually be cooked. They normally cook in 8–10 minutes. Check by breaking a noodle in half – it is cooked when it is the same colour right through to the centre. Drain and rinse in cold water before serving.

Pasta with Vegetable Sauce

Ideal for a light lunch or evening snack.

SERVES 4

4 cups (700g/1½lb) cooked pasta	50g (2oz) cauliflower florets
1 tablespoon toasted sesame oil	a pinch of sea salt
1 onion, peeled, halved and sliced	1–2 tablespoons shoyu

2 carrots, scrubbed and diced

1 leek, split, washed and cut into 1cm
 (¼in) slices

100g (4oz) broccoli florets

½ cup (75g/3oz) sweetcorn kernels

peas or sliced green beans

1 tablespoon mirin *or* 2 teaspoons
 ginger juice (see page 75)

½–1 tablespoon kuzu

a few slices of lemon

some chopped parsley or finely sliced
 spring onion

1. Heat the toasted sesame oil in a pan and sauté the onion for 3–4 minutes. Add the other vegetables, 2 cups (500ml/¾ pint) water and a pinch of salt, and cook in a covered pan until the vegetables are just soft. Add the shoyu and mirin or ginger juice, and thicken the liquid with a little kuzu dissolved in cold water.

2. Put the cooked pasta into a serving dish and pour the sauce over. Garnish with a few slices of lemon and some chopped parsley or sliced spring onions, and serve hot.

VARIATION

Alternatively, you can make the dish as above, varying the vegetables according to what you have available, then place the pasta in a heatproof dish and cover with plenty of sauce. Bake at 180°C/350°F/Gas Mark 4 for 20–30 minutes. When cooked, sprinkle some lemon juice over. Garnish with lots of chopped parsley or finely sliced spring onions.

Fried Udon Noodles ◎

The toasted sunflower seeds add flavour and a lovely crunchy texture.

SERVES 3–4

1 x 200g (7oz) packet Udon noodles

1 tablespoon toasted sesame oil

2 onions, peeled and finely sliced

1 clove garlic, peeled and crushed
 (optional)

2 carrots, scrubbed and cut into
 matchsticks

2 sticks celery, finely sliced

6 mushrooms, wiped and finely sliced

a little shoyu

1 tablespoon mirin

2 teaspoons ginger juice (see page 75)

2 tablespoons lightly toasted sunflower
 seeds

2 spring onions, finely sliced

1. Bring 8 cups (2 litres/3½ pints) water to the boil in a large saucepan and add the noodles, a few at a time, stirring to prevent sticking. There is no need to add salt as the noodles already contain some. Bring back to the boil and simmer until expanded and fully cooked. You can tell when the noodles are cooked by breaking one in half. They should be the same colour right through to the centre. Place them in a colander, rinse under cold water and drain thoroughly.

2. Next, heat the oil in a large pan or wok and add the onions. Sauté until soft and translucent before adding the garlic (if using). Continue to cook for about 2 minutes, stirring all the time, before adding the carrots, celery and mushrooms. Sauté for 2–3 minutes, then add a small cup (150ml/5fl oz) water, plus the shoyu and mirin.

3. Place the cooked noodles on top of the vegetables. Cover and simmer for 5 minutes. Sprinkle the ginger juice over the noodles and cook for 1 further minute.
4. Transfer to a serving dish, then stir in the sunflower seeds, garnish with the spring onion and serve.

VARIATIONS

This recipe also works really well with leftover brown rice. Replace the noodles with 2–3 cups (350–500g/ 12oz–1lb 2oz) cooked rice and proceed as before. Also, if you are unable to get genuine, quality Japanese Udon noodles, you can use your favourite spaghetti or similar pasta.

YIN *Pasta Salad with Smoked Tofu*

A wonderfully colourful salad with a fresh taste.

SERVES 4–6

175g (6oz) wholewheat pasta shapes

a pinch of sea salt

2 carrots, scrubbed and diced

175g (6oz) broccoli florets

1 x 225g (8oz) block smoked tofu, cubed

12 radishes, halved

12 black olives (optional)

1 tablespoon chopped parsley

Dressing

2–3 tablespoons shoyu

1 tablespoon grain mustard

2 tablespoons toasted sesame seed oil

2–3 tablespoons cider vinegar *or*

brown rice vinegar

1. Cook the pasta in plenty of boiling water with a pinch of salt for about 10 minutes or according to the instructions on the packet. Place in a colander, rinse under cold water and drain thoroughly.
2. Cook the carrots and broccoli in a pan of boiling water with a pinch of salt for 1–2 minutes. Remove from the pan, refresh under the cold water tap and drain. Place the pasta, carrots, broccoli, tofu, radishes and olives (if using) in a large serving bowl.
3. Put all the dressing ingredients into a bowl and whisk until well mixed. Pour over the salad and toss together. Sprinkle with the parsley and serve.

VARIATION

Pan-fry the tofu in a little good oil and drain on kitchen paper before adding to the salad.

BEANS, TOFU AND TEMPEH

Beans

You can use any type of bean – aduki, chickpeas, haricot, mung, kidney or pinto beans – in this recipe.

SERVES 2–3

1 cup (175g/6oz) beans

1 x 8cm (3in) piece of kombu

1 teaspoon shoyu *or* pinch of sea salt

1. Pick over the beans carefully to get rid of stones or grit, and wash. Soak in 3 cups (750ml/1¼ pints) water for 6–8 hours. Alternatively, you can reduce the soaking time to 4 hours by soaking them in boiling water. Soaking makes the beans easier to cook and much more digestible when cooked thoroughly.
2. Transfer them to a pan with the kombu and soaking water and bring to the boil. Simmer for 10 minutes, remove any foam that forms and cover with a lid. Cook until quite soft – usually 1–2 hours, depending on the type of bean. Remove the lid and add the shoyu or salt. Simmer, uncovered, for 5 minutes. During the cooking you can add more cold water if needed.
3. You can also pressure-cook the beans, releasing the pressure to season and continuing to cook without pressure until the liquid has almost gone. Never add

salt or soy sauce until the beans have softened. If you
add it too soon, the beans may not soften at all. Use the
cooked beans in your favourite dishes or in the following recipes.

YIN **Bean Salad**

Mix cooked beans with a selection of contrasting colour
vegetables (cut small, lightly boiled and still crunchy) and
add some raw, chopped spring onions. Make a tasty dressing, such as Lemon (page 133), Mustard (page 134) or
Herb (page 132), or be inventive and make up your own.
This is delicious served with noodles.

YIN **Hummus**

*Serve this on bread, ricecakes or stuffed into some pitta breads with
some green salad, pickled gherkins, lemon wedges and parsley.*

SERVES 4–6

2 cups (400g/14oz) cooked chickpeas	1 dessertspoon umeboshi paste
or 425g tin of organic chickpeas	1 dessertspoon grain mustard
drained	1–2 dessertspoons tahini
1 clove garlic, peeled (optional)	1–2 dessertspoons lemon juice

1. Put all the ingredients in a blender and whizz together,
adding a little cold water if needed.

Simple Bean Stew

An easy and satisfying meal.

SERVES 2–3

1 tablespoon sesame oil

1 onion, peeled and diced

1 large carrot, scrubbed and diced

1 cup (200g/7oz) cooked chickpeas (or
other beans)

1 tablespoon shoyu

1–2 teaspoons of ginger juice
(see page 75)

1 dessertspoon kuzu

some chopped parsley

1. Heat the oil in a pan, sauté the onion until soft and then add the carrot. Sauté for a couple of minutes, then add the chickpeas, any cooking liquid and, if necessary, some cold water to give a stew-like consistency.
2. Simmer until the vegetables are soft and add the shoyu and ginger juice. Continue simmering for a further 4 minutes, then thicken slightly with the kuzu (dissolved in a little cold water).
3. Serve garnished with the chopped parsley.

YIN   ## Barbecued Beans

Perfect on their own or placed (covered) in a medium oven for 15 minutes to make baked beans (which are more Yang).

SERVES 4–6

2 cups (350g/12oz) haricot beans

1 x 8cm (3in) strip of kombu, wiped

2 bay leaves

2 sticks celery, sliced

2–3 tablespoons shoyu

2 tablespoons rice syrup or barley malt

1 tablespoon sesame oil

2 small onions, peeled and sliced

2 cloves garlic, peeled and minced
 (optional)

1 teaspoon ground cumin (optional)

1 teaspoon ground coriander (optional)

2 carrots, scrubbed and diced

3 tablespoons rice vinegar or cider
 vinegar

2 teaspoons ginger juice (see page 75)

1–2 tablespoons arrowroot or kuzu
 (optional)

some chopped parsley

1. Pick over and rinse the haricot beans. Then soak them in 4 cups (1 litre/1¾ pints) water for 4 hours.

2. Place the kombu in a heavy saucepan and cover with the beans and soaking liquid. Bring to the boil, uncovered, and simmer for 10 minutes, skimming off any foam. Add the bay leaves, cover and cook until the beans are soft (about 1–1½ hours).

3. Meanwhile, heat the oil in a saucepan and add the onion and garlic. Sauté gently for 3 or 4 minutes. Add the cumin and coriander (if using) and stir for 1–2 minutes. Add a little water, the carrots and celery, then bring to the boil, cover and simmer until the vegetables are just soft.

4. Now add the cooked beans and kombu (sliced) to the vegetables and enough of the cooking liquid to reach just below the level of the beans. Stir in the shoyu, rice syrup or barley malt and vinegar, and simmer for 5 minutes. Add the ginger juice to the pan and simmer for another 2 minutes.

5. If the sauce is too runny, thicken it with arrowroot or kuzu dissolved in a little cold water. Add this to the

bean liquid and stir for 1–2 minutes. Serve garnished with parsley.

Bean Croquettes

These are also popular shaped into burgers for children.

SERVES 3–4

a little olive oil	1 tablespoon tahini
1 onion, peeled and diced	1 teaspoon grain mustard
1 clove garlic, peeled and minced	1 teaspoon dried mixed herbs
1 carrot, scrubbed and finely grated	sea salt or shoyu and freshly ground
a few drops of shoyu	black pepper to taste
1 cup (200g/7oz) cooked beans (e.g.	plain wholemeal flour
chickpeas, kidney beans,	oil for frying
butterbeans or lentils)	

1. Heat the olive oil in a pan and sauté the onion for about 5 minutes without browning. Add the garlic, carrot and shoyu and continue to sauté for a further 5 minutes.
2. Mash the cooked beans until fairly smooth, then add the sautéed vegetables and the tahini, mustard, herbs and seasonings. Mix thoroughly together. Add the flour, a tablespoon at a time (about 2–3 tablespoons to make a fairly stiff mix). You can add a little bean cooking liquid or cold water to get it to bind if necessary.

3. Place the bean mixture in a covered bowl in the refrigerator for about half an hour to firm up and then make
into small balls or croquettes. Moisten or flour your
hands to stop the mixture sticking. Use about a soup
spoon full of mixture for each ball. Place the croquettes
on a floured plate or tray. Heat some oil in a pan and
fry gently until golden brown, turning once. If they
splatter, coat them in some flour before frying but do
not have the oil too hot or the flour will burn. Drain on
kitchen paper.

4. Serve with a tangy chutney or sauce, or Tahini and
Lemon Dip (see page 134).

VARIATIONS
You can try using different vegetables in these bean
croquettes – mushrooms, celery, red peppers, plus your
favourite seasonings. They are delicious with sweetcorn
kernels added and shaped into burgers and served in pitta
breads with salad, coleslaw and pickles. Be creative!
Instead of frying, place them on a lightly oiled baking
tray and bake at 350°C/180°F/Gas Mark 4 for about 20
minutes.

Baked Stuffed Pumpkin

Full of flavour and great for a Hallowe'en feast!

SERVES 4–6

1 x 1.5kg (3lb) pumpkin

50g (2oz) shelled walnuts, washed

1 tablespoon sesame oil

1 onion, peeled and diced

1 carrot, scrubbed and diced

2 sticks celery, sliced

6 mushrooms, wiped and chopped

2 tablespoons shoyu

3 tablespoons dry couscous (or any cooked grain)

125g (4oz) plain tofu, mashed

1/2 teaspoon dried thyme

a pinch of sea salt

freshly ground black pepper to taste (optional)

1. Slice the top off the pumpkin and scoop out the seeds. Place the top and base in a pan with 2.5cm (1in) boiling water and steam for about 15 minutes until beginning to turn soft. Remove carefully and leave to cool a little.
2. Roast the walnuts in the oven at 350°C/180°F/Gas Mark 4 for 5–7 minutes. Break into quarters or chop.
3. Heat the oil in a pan and sauté the onion until soft. Add the carrot, celery and mushrooms and sauté for 2–3 minutes. Add the shoyu and 1 cup (250ml/8fl oz) water and simmer, covered, for 10 minutes. Add the couscous, stir, cover again, and leave to stand for 5 minutes.
4. Stir in the walnuts, tofu, thyme, salt and black pepper. Then stuff the mixture well down into the pumpkin base and replace the top. Place in a baking dish and bake in a preheated oven at 200°C/400°F/Gas Mark 6 for 30 minutes.

YIN   ## *Tofu Cheese*   ◎

A wonderful alternative to full-fat cheese especially if you have an intolerance for dairy products.

SERVES 2–4

1 x 200g (7oz) block plain tofu   1–2 teaspoons ginger juice (see page 75)

50g (2oz) shelled walnuts, washed   2 spring onions, finely sliced

1 dessertspoon mugi miso

1. Boil the tofu for 2 minutes in plain water and drain.
2. Roast the walnuts on a tray in the oven at 180°C/350°F/Gas Mark 4 until evenly roasted (5–7 minutes). Grind nuts finely and blend in the tofu. Add the miso and ginger juice to your taste and blend.
3. Mix in the spring onions and serve on your favourite crackers, crispbread or rolls.

VARIATION

Try serving as an appetiser, spread on halves of ricecake with a little green salad, thin slices of red pepper or some grated carrot and a few good olives.

Baked Tofu

Tofu is an excellent source of protein — perfect for vegetarians.

SERVES 4

1 tablespoon sunflower oil

2 onions, peeled and thinly sliced

2 carrots, scrubbed, halved and thinly
 sliced or ½ small pumpkin, peeled,
 de-seeded and cubed

1–2 tablespoons tahini or peanut butter

1–2 tablespoons miso

2 tablespoons lemon juice

200g (7oz) block plain tofu

chopped parsley, sliced spring
 onion or a few lemon wedges
 (optional)

1. Heat the oil and sauté the onions until translucent. Add the carrots or pumpkin and a little water and simmer until the vegetables are just soft.
2. Remove from the heat, mash well and mix with a purée made from the tahini or peanut butter, miso, lemon juice and some of the cooking liquid or extra water.
3. Cut the tofu into about eight slices and arrange them on a baking tray or ovenproof dish. Pour the sauce over them, ensuring that all the pieces of tofu are evenly coated, and bake at 180°C/350°F/Gas Mark 4 for about 20 minutes. Garnish with parsley, spring onion or lemon wedges if you wish.

Scrambled Tofu

SERVES 3–4

1 tablespoon sunflower or sesame oil

1 onion, peeled and diced

6–8 mushrooms, wiped and chopped

sweetcorn kernels from 1 corn cob

1 x 200g (7oz) plain or smoked tofu

2 teaspoons shoyu

1 sheet nori

2 spring onions, finely sliced

1. Heat the oil in a pan and sauté the onion until soft. Add the mushrooms and sweetcorn. Crumble the tofu and add, mixing thoroughly. Add a little cold water and the shoyu and simmer for 5 minutes. Break the nori into small pieces, and stir in to the mixture.
2. Serve on sourdough bread with some finely sliced spring onions for garnish.

VARIATIONS

You can add a little black pepper to the mixture if you like or spread a thin layer of grain mustard on the bread.

Tofu and Vegetable Flan

Delicious served warm or cold.

SERVES 4–6

150g (5oz) wholemeal pastry flour (fine)

sea salt

50 ml (2fl oz) corn oil or sunflower oil

1 tablespoon olive oil

2 onions, peeled and sliced

1 x 225g (8oz) block regular tofu

1 dessertspoon grain mustard

1 tablespoon shoyu

1 teaspoon dried marjoram (or other herb)

2 tablespoons sweetcorn kernels

100g (4oz) small cauliflower florets

freshly ground black pepper to taste

(optional)

1. Preheat oven to 190°C/375°F/Gas Mark 5.

2. First prepare the pastry by mixing the flour with a pinch of salt and rubbing in the corn or sunflower oil very gently until you get a crumb texture. Add enough cold water (about 3–5 tablespoons) to make a soft dough which comes away from the sides of the bowl, but do not over-mix. Lightly oil a 20cm (8in) flan tin and then roll out the pastry on a floured board until it is large enough to fill the base. Place in the tin and prick the base all over with a fork.

3. Meanwhile, heat the olive oil in a pan and sauté the onions until soft. Add the sweetcorn and the cauliflower, a pinch of sea salt and about ½ cup (85ml/3fl oz) water. Cover the pan and simmer for about 5 minutes.

4. Drain the vegetables and add the cooking liquid to the tofu in a large bowl, together with the mustard, shoyu, dried herbs and pepper. Whizz the tofu mixture in the blender until soft and creamy (adding a little extra water if needed), and mix with the vegetables.

5. Fill the pastry case and smooth over. Place in the middle of the oven and bake for 35–40 minutes or until golden brown all over and fairly well set. Remove from the oven and allow to stand for at least 15 minutes before serving.

YIN   *Marinated Vegetable Kebabs*
       with Smoked Tofu

Excellent as a main course or serves 8 as a snack or party food.

SERVES 4

16 carrot slices, about 1cm (¼in) thick	1 dessertspoon mirin
16 broccoli florets	1 tablespoon ginger juice (see page 75)
8 button mushrooms, wiped	1 x 225g (8oz) block smoked tofu, cut
sea salt	into 16 cubes
2 tablespoons shoyu	

1. Blanch the vegetables very lightly for 1–2 minutes in boiling water with a pinch of salt. Rinse in cold water and drain.
2. Make a marinade with the shoyu, mirin, ginger juice and 4 tablespoons cold water. Let the vegetables and tofu soak in the mixture for at least an hour, stirring occasionally.
3. Drain and divide equally between 8 kebab sticks. Strain the remaining marinade and serve as a dip in a separate bowl.

VARIATIONS

You can use regular unsmoked tofu instead, preferably boiled for 2 minutes before marinating. For another variation, grill or barbecue the marinated kebabs before serving with the dip.

YANG *Deep-fried Tofu and Winter Vegetable Stew*

Flavour and texture are all-important in this highly nutritious dish.

SERVES 4

1 x 5cm (2in) strip of kombu

2 onions, peeled and quartered

2 carrots, scrubbed and cut into 2.5cm (1in) chunks

225g (8oz) pumpkin, peeled and cut into 2.5cm (1in) chunks

1 x 225g (8oz) block deep-fried tofu, cubed

1–2 tablespoons shoyu

1–2 teaspoons ginger juice (see page 75)

2 teaspoons kuzu or arrowroot

2 spring onions, finely sliced

1. Soak the kombu in 3–4fl oz water for 10 minutes, then finely slice.
2. Place the kombu and its soaking liquid in the bottom of a heavy pan and add the onions, followed by the carrots and pumpkin. Barely cover with cold water and bring to the boil. Cover and simmer for 10 minutes.
3. Add the tofu and continue to cook, covered, until the vegetables are just soft. Add the shoyu and ginger juice and simmer, uncovered, for a further 2 minutes.
4. Dilute the kuzu or arrowroot in a little cold water and add to the stew. Stir gently until the sauce has thickened. Serve garnished with the sliced spring onions.

YANG   ## Seitan Stew with Pumpkin and Leeks

This is a wonderful vegetable casserole.

SERVES 4

1 tablespoon toasted sesame oil	1 tablespoon shoyu
2 leeks, thinly sliced	1 dessertspoon grain mustard
½ small pumpkin, peeled, de-seeded and cubed	1–2 teaspoons kuzu
	some chopped parsley
1 x 200g (8oz) pack ready-cooked seitan	

1. Heat the oil in a deep pan and sauté the leeks until they are soft but not browned. Place the pumpkin chunks on top of the leeks, then cut the seitan into chunks and put this on top of the pumpkin. Add enough cold water to half-cover the pumpkin, bring to the boil and simmer, covered, until the pumpkin is soft.
2. Add the shoyu and mustard, stir well and simmer for a further 5 minutes. If necessary, thicken the liquid with kuzu dissolved in a little cold water. Place in a bowl, garnish with the parsley and serve.

Fried Tempeh with Ginger Sauce

Serve the tempeh on cocktail sticks with the sauce in a bowl for dipping, or add the tempeh to the sauce, heat through and serve as a stew over your favourite grain dish.

SERVES 4

1 x 8cm (3in) strip of kombu	2 tablespoons shoyu
3–4 slices fresh ginger	1 x 227g (8oz) block tempeh, thawed
1–2 teaspoons ginger juice (see page 75)	oil for frying
2 cloves garlic, peeled and sliced	2 tablespoons barley malt or rice syrup
1 bay leaf	1–2 tablespoons kuzu or arrowroot

1. Put 600ml (1 pint) cold water in a pan and add the kombu, ginger slices, garlic, bay leaf and shoyu. Bring to the boil and add the block of tempeh. Reduce the heat to a simmer, cover the pan and cook for 20 minutes.
2. Remove the tempeh from the stock, drain and pat dry. Cut into 16 squares. Heat the oil in a pan and fry the tempeh pieces until golden brown. Remove and drain.
3. Strain the cooking liquid and add the barley malt or rice syrup to it, plus extra soy sauce if needed. Add the ginger juice into the liquid. Bring the mixture to a simmer and dissolve the kuzu or arrowroot in a little cold water. Stir this in until the mixture thickens slightly.

FISH

@

YANG   *Smoked Mackerel Pâté*

This can also be used as a sandwich-filler with a crunchy salad.

SERVES 6–8 AS A STARTER OR SNACK

½ x 225g (8oz) block plain tofu   1 dessertspoon grain mustard

2 small fillets of smoked mackerel   chopped parsley

1 small onion, peeled and diced   lemon wedges

1 dessertspoon tahini (optional)

1. Boil the tofu in water for 2 minutes and leave to drain.
2. Skin the fillets of mackerel and break up with a fork. Place the mackerel, tofu, onion, tahini (if using) and mustard in a blender and whizz until smooth. Add a little water if necessary.
3. Serve on crackers or sourdough bread with parsley and lemon wedges.

⊚ YANG   *Roasted Cod with Wasabi and Parsley Topping*

Eating fish two or three times a week will give you an optimal amount of nutrients.

SERVES 4

1 small onion, peeled and finely diced

2 carrots, scrubbed and cut into matchsticks

4 x 110g (4oz) fillets of cod, skinned

1 tablespoon chopped parsley

1–2 teaspoons wasabi powder *or* 1 dessertspoon grain mustard

1 lemon, scrubbed and halved

1 tablespoon olive oil

1/4 teaspoon sea salt

freshly ground black pepper to taste

some extra chopped parsley

1. Spread the onion and carrots on an oiled baking tray, then lay the fish on top.
2. Place the parsley, wasabi or mustard, 1 tablespoon of juice from half a lemon, olive oil, salt and some black pepper in a bowl and mix together. Spread the mixture over the fish.
3. Roast in a preheated oven at 190°C/375°F/Gas Mark 5 for about 10 minutes, until the fish is just cooked through. Remove from the oven and carefully place the fish and vegetables on a warm plate. Garnish with the parsley and the remaining lemon half, sliced.

YANG · **Baked Herring** ◎

Herring is high in Omega 3 — an essential fat which protects against heart disease.

SERVES 2

1 dessertspoon shoyu

1 tablespoon lemon juice

2 small herring fillets

lemon wedges, parsley sprigs and 1 tablespoon raw, grated daikon or radish to
 garnish

1. Preheat oven to 190°C/375°F/Gas Mark 5.
2. Mix the shoyu and lemon juice in a shallow baking dish and add the fish. Coat well with the marinade and let stand for 10 minutes.
3. Place in the oven and bake for about 10 minutes until the fish is just cooked through. Serve garnished with lemon wedges, parsley and grated daikon or radish.

VARIATIONS

You can also try trout or mackerel in this recipe.

YANG   *Haddock with White Sauce*

SERVES 2

1 onion, finely sliced in half moons

1 tablespoon mirin

1 teaspoon wholegrain mustard

2 small haddock fillets

1 tablespoon white miso

1 tablespoon kuzu

a few sprigs of parsley, lemon wedges

and 1 tablespoon raw grated daikon

or radish to garnish

1. Place 150ml (¼ pint) water in a wide saucepan and bring to the boil. Add the onion slices and simmer, covered, on a gentle flame for 10 minutes until quite soft. Add the mirin and mustard and stir.
2. Gently lay the fish on top of the onions in the pan and cover. Cook slowly for about 8 minutes until the fish is just beginning to flake.
3. Remove the fish and onions from the pan and place on a heated serving dish. Return the pan with the remaining liquid to the heat and stir in the white miso. Dissolve the kuzu in a little cold water and add to the pan, stirring all the time. As soon as the sauce thickens, remove from the heat and pour over the fish. Garnish with parsley, lemon wedges and raw, grated daikon or radish.

VARIATION

You can also use cod or plaice for this recipe. The cooking time will depend on the thickness of the fish and will need to be adjusted accordingly.

VEGETABLES

YIN   ## *Pressed Salad*

Try one of the dressings on pages 132–4 instead of adding brown rice vinegar.

SERVES 6

1 cucumber, finely sliced	1 tablespoon dulse, finely chopped
a bunch of radishes, finely sliced	1/2–1 tablespoon brown rice vinegar
2 sticks celery, finely sliced	some chopped parsley
1 teaspoon sea salt	

1. Place the vegetables in a bowl or pickle press and mix with the salt. Cover with a plate and a heavy weight or press in the pickle press and leave for about 2 hours.
2. Meanwhile, check the dulse for stones and shells, rinse and soak in a very small amount of cold water for 5 minutes. Drain and squeeze out the extra moisture (use for soup stock or to water houseplants).
3. Place the vegetables in a colander to drain thoroughly, rinsing if too salty. Add the dulse and rice vinegar, mix together and garnish with some parsley if you wish. The salad will keep in the fridge, covered, for 2–3 days.

VARIATIONS

Alternatively, use grated carrot with finely sliced celery, Chinese leaf and very finely sliced radishes. For the dressing, you can use soy sauce with lemon juice, umeboshi vinegar with rice vinegar, or cider vinegar with salt or shoyu.

127

YANG *Nishime Steamed Vegetables*

Steaming creates soft, juicy vegetables.

SERVES

1 x 8cm (3in) strip of kombu	a pinch of sea salt
a selection of vegetables	soy sauce to taste
(e.g.carrots and onions, pumpkins	mirin *or* ginger juice (see page 75) to taste
and onions, daikon, cabbage, swede,	a little kuzu
turnip and burdock)	some chopped parsley

1. Soak the kombu in a little water for 10 minutes, then cut into very thin strips.
2. Cut the vegetables into large chunks. Place the kombu in the bottom of a cast iron pan and layer the vegetables on top, starting with the softest and finishing with the hardest (e.g. carrots on top of onions). Add the kombu soaking liquid and enough water to half cover the vegetables, add a pinch of salt, cover and bring to the boil. Turn down the heat and cook for about 20 minutes until the vegetables are almost soft (try not to keep removing the lid – it is better left alone).
3. Now season with the soy sauce and mirin or ginger juice, cover and shake the pan carefully and allow to simmer for a further 5 minutes.
4. If there is still some liquid in the pan, thicken it with a small amount of kuzu (diluted in cold water), and pour over the vegetables as a glaze. Garnish with a little chopped parsley, and serve.

YIN   **Green Sauerkraut Rolls**   @

A good alternative for party snacks or a light lunch.

ONE LARGE LEAF SERVES 2–3
some large spring green leaves
sauerkraut

1. Boil the green leaves whole until they are very dark green and just beginning to soften. Drain and cool thoroughly, cut out the stems and place the leaves on a sushi mat.
2. Place 1–2 tablespoons drained sauerkraut in a sausage shape about 2.5cm (1in) from the bottom end of the leaf. Carefully roll up like a rice sushi and squeeze gently to remove any excess juice. Remove from the sushi mat and slice into circles about 2.5cm (1in) thick. Serve cut end up.

YIN   **Boiled Salad**

Choose a selection of vegetables from the following combinations.

- 0.25cm (¼in) rounds carrot, thin rings or half moons onion and 0.25cm (¼in) slices celery
- halved radishes, 0.25cm (¼in) half rounds cucumber and small florets cauliflower
- 0.25cm (¼in) half rounds daikon (mooli), small florets broccoli or shredded red cabbage

🌀 **1.** Lightly boil or blanch the vegetables with a pinch of sea salt and drain well. They should normally only need about 1–2 minutes, depending on their size. Serve with a dressing of your choice (see pages 132–4).

YIN *Cauliflower, Broccoli and Carrot Salad*

SERVES 3–4

110g (4oz) broccoli florets

110g (4oz) cauliflower florets

2 large carrots, scrubbed, halved lengthways and sliced

a pinch of sea salt

1. Boil each vegetable separately in lightly salted boiling water for 2–3 minutes. As each one is removed from the pot, refresh it in a colander under a cold running tap.

2. Drain the vegetables and place together in a serving dish. Toss in the dressing of your choice. The Sweet and Sour Dulse Dressing (see page 133) is particularly good with this.

YIN *Sweetcorn, Carrot and Green Bean Salad*

SERVES 3–4

sweetcorn kernels from 2 corn cobs

220g (8oz) green beans, trimmed and sliced

2 large carrots, scrubbed and cut into matchsticks

1. Prepare as in the previous recipe, but cook the beans a little longer and the sweetcorn a little less.

YIN ## *Steamed Greens*

SERVES 3–4

A selection of green leaves (e.g. cabbage, spring greens, Chinese leaf and
 watercress)

1. Slice the greens into strips and steam for 2–3 minutes. The greens can be steamed in a suspended basket or covered colander or you can place them in a small amount of boiling water in a lidded saucepan.
2. Cool quickly on a large plate or tray and toss in a dressing of your choice such as Mustard Dressing (page 134) or Lemon Dressing (page 133), just before serving.

Arame Stir-fry

Arame is high in iron and calcium – I love it best cooked with a selection of crunchy vegetables.

SERVES 4

25g (1oz) arame	1 small red pepper, de-seeded and
1 tablespoon sesame oil	diced
1 clove garlic, peeled and minced	110g (4oz) small broccoli florets
2 teaspoons grated fresh ginger	2 tablespoons shoyu
2 onions, peeled and finely sliced	2 tablespoons sunflower seeds, lightly
2 carrots, scrubbed and cut into	toasted
matchsticks	3 spring onions, finely sliced

1. Rinse the arame in a sieve under a cold tap, drain, place in a bowl, cover with cold water and soak for 15 minutes.

2. Heat the oil in a wok or large, deep frying pan and add the garlic and grated ginger. Stir-fry for a minute and then add the onions. Cook for 2 minutes before adding the carrots. Continue stir-frying for a further 2 minutes, then add the soaked arame, red pepper and broccoli florets, plus any liquid from the arame or about 2 tablespoons of water. Add the shoyu, mix thoroughly, cover and cook gently for 3 minutes.

3. Remove from the heat, mix in the toasted sunflower seeds and sliced spring onion, and serve immediately.

DRESSINGS AND SAUCES

YIN
Herb Dressing

Quick and simple to make.

SERVES 4

2 tablespoons olive oil *or* toasted sesame oil

2 tablespoons cider vinegar *or* brown rice vinegar

1 clove garlic, peeled and crushed (optional)

sea salt and freshly ground black pepper to taste

1 tablespoon freshly chopped herbs (e.g. parsley, basil, chives or dill)

1. Place the oil, vinegar and garlic (if using) in a bowl and whisk to emulsify. Add seasoning to taste and whisk

again. Stir in the herbs and serve. Or refrigerate in a ◉
screw-top jar until required.

YIN ## Lemon Dressing

SERVES 4

2 tablespoons olive oil or toasted sesame oil
juice of 1 lemon
1 tablespoon shoyu

1. Place all the ingredients in a bowl with 2–4 tablespoons cold water and whisk together. Use immediately or store as for Herb Dressing (above).

YIN ## Sweet and Sour Dulse Dressing

This dressing is excellent with lightly boiled or steamed vegetables,
particularly cauliflower and broccoli.

SERVES 4

1 tablespoon dulse	1 tablespoon ume plum seasoning
2 tablespoons toasted sesame oil	1 tablespoon brown rice vinegar
1–2 tablespoons barley malt or	1 spring onion, finely sliced
brown rice syrup	

1. Check the dulse for stones or shells, then rinse and
   soak in a little cold water for 5 minutes. Drain and chop
   finely.

133

2. Place all the ingredients in a bowl with 2 tablespoons cold water, mix thoroughly, and allow to stand for 10 minutes before serving.

YIN **Mustard Dressing**

SERVES 4

2 tablespoons toasted sesame oil or olive oil

1 tablespoon cider vinegar or brown rice vinegar

2 teaspoons grain mustard

1 tablespoon shoyu

1 tablespoon chopped parsley

1. Blend the oil, vinegar, mustard and shoyu together with 1–2 tablespoons cold water. Stir in the parsley just before serving.

YIN **Tahini and Lemon Dip**

Dips are easy to create and make a healthy snack.

SERVES 4

3 tablespoons tahini

juice of 1 lemon

sea salt and freshly ground black pepper to taste

1 tablespoon chopped parsley

1. Blend the tahini with the lemon juice and 2 tablespoons cold water. Season with salt and pepper, add the parsley, and serve.

Carrot and Nut Dip

*Serve with your favourite bread or a selection of colourful crudités
and pitta breads or corn nachos.*

SERVES 4

1 onion, peeled and thinly sliced

450g (1lb) carrots, scrubbed and thinly sliced

1 tablespoon almond butter *or* hazelnut butter (see Glossary)

2 teaspoons shoyu

1. Place the onion in a saucepan with the carrots on top
   and add 1 cup (175ml/6fl oz) water and a pinch of salt.
   Bring to the boil, cover and simmer until soft (about
   15–20 minutes). (Or you can cook the vegetables in a
   pressure cooker which will only take 5–7 minutes.)
2. Remove the vegetables from the pan and drain, reserving the cooking liquor for stock. Blend the vegetables
   to a purée with the nut butter and shoyu, adding a little
   of the cooking liquor if needed to obtain a dip consistency.

VARIATION

You can make this dip richer by adding more nut butter –
up to double the amount.

Lentil Sauce

SERVES 4

1 cup (175g/6oz) puy or green lentils	1 bay leaf
1 tablespoon sunflower oil	1 teaspoon dried thyme
2 onions, peeled and diced	1 x 12cm (5in) piece of wakame
1 clove garlic, peeled and crushed	1–2 tablespoons barley miso
2 sticks celery, thinly sliced	small piece of fresh ginger, washed
2 carrots, scrubbed and diced	a little kuzu or arrowroot (optional)

1. Pick over, wash and drain the lentils.
2. Heat the oil in a saucepan and add the onions, stirring continually until they begin to soften. Add the garlic and stir for a further 1–2 minutes, then take the pan off the heat. Now add the celery, carrots, bay leaf, thyme and 600ml (1 pint) water.
3. Rinse the wakame and soak in a little cold water for a few minutes until soft enough to slice into small pieces. Add with the soaking water to the pan, then cover with the lentils. Bring to the boil, skim off any foam, reduce the flame, cover and simmer until the lentils are soft – about 30–40 minutes.
4. Add the miso, puréed in a little of the cooking liquid, and continue to simmer very gently for 3–4 minutes. Grate some ginger root, squeeze the juice into the lentils and allow to cook for just 1–2 minutes longer.
5. If you require a thicker consistency dissolve some kuzu or arrowroot in a little cold water and stir into the lentils.

Mushroom Sauce

Delicious served on your favourite pasta or with couscous.

SERVES 3–4

4 dried shiitake mushrooms

1 x 7cm (3in) strip of kombu

1 tablespoon sesame oil

1 onion, peeled, halved and sliced

1 clove garlic, peeled and crushed

 (optional)

12 fresh mushrooms, wiped and thinly

 sliced

2–3 tablespoons shoyu

freshly ground black pepper to taste

a little kuzu or arrowroot

1 tablespoon chopped parsley

1. Soak the shiitake mushrooms in 90–120ml (3–4fl oz) hot water for 30 minutes. Drain, reserving the soaking liquid, then discard the shiitake stalks and slice the tops finely.

2. Soak the kombu in 90–120ml (3–4fl oz) cold water for 5 minutes. Then drain, reserving the soaking liquid.

3. Place the sliced shiitake mushrooms in a saucepan with the kombu and all the soaking liquids. Then add enough cold water to make the total quantity of liquid up to about 300ml (½ pint). Bring to the boil and simmer for 5–6 minutes. Remove the pan from the heat and take out the kombu (store in the fridge for future use).

4. In a separate pan, heat the oil and sauté the onion and garlic until soft. Add the fresh mushrooms and stir for a couple of minutes. Add the mushroom, kombu stock and sliced shiitake tops, bring to the boil and simmer,

covered, for about 10 minutes. Add the shoyu and some black pepper and simmer, uncovered, for 2 minutes.

5. Dilute a little kuzu or arrowroot in cold water and stir into the sauce to thicken. Garnish with parsley and serve immediately.

SWEET THINGS

YIN

Ginger Apricots with Toasted Almonds

A truly wonderful combination of flavours.

SERVES 6

225g (8oz) dried unsulphured, stoned apricots

a pinch of sea salt

about 18 whole almonds

a small piece of fresh ginger

kuzu (optional)

1. Rinse the apricots in warm water, place in a saucepan with the salt and cover with cold water. Bring to the boil, reduce the heat, cover and simmer until the fruit is very soft. Add more cold water from time to time if needed.
2. Meanwhile, place the almonds on a tray and roast them in the oven at 180°C/350°F/Gas Mark 4 for 5 minutes. Then shake them and roast for a further 2–3 minutes. Remove from the oven and allow to cool.
3. When the fruit is soft, grate the ginger root and

squeeze over the fruit, extracting the juice (you need 2–3 teaspoons). Add a little kuzu dissolved in cold water to thicken if too runny. Simmer for 1 minute and remove from heat.

4. Serve hot or cold, garnished with the whole almonds.

YIN ## *Apple and Almond Mousse*

Amasake can be used for many delicious desserts.

SERVES 6–8

1 x 380g (13oz) jar amasake (see Glossary)	50g (2oz) ground almonds
350ml (12fl oz) apple juice	2 dessertspoons kuzu
a pinch of sea salt	a few drops of almond essence (optional)
4 heaped dessertspoons of agar agar flakes	a few roasted whole almonds to garnish

1. Mix the amasake and apple juice together with the salt and agar agar flakes in a pan and leave to stand for 10 minutes. Place on the heat and bring to a gentle simmer, stirring regularly. Allow to simmer for about 5 minutes to dissolve the agar flakes.

2. Add the ground almonds to the mixture. Dissolve the kuzu with a little cold water, then stir into the amasake mixture until it thickens slightly. Add the almond essence, stir in thoroughly and transfer to a shallow, moistened dish to cool for an hour.

3. Blend or whisk the pudding and leave to set again

(this takes about 1 hour) in a moistened mould or in individual dishes. Garnish with whole almonds and serve.

YIN *Fruit Custard*

A new twist on an old favourite.

SERVES 4–6

110g (4oz) raisins	600ml (1 pint) soy milk
a pinch of sea salt	½ teaspoon vanilla essence
1 apple, finely sliced	1 tablespoon rice syrup
1 pear, finely sliced	a little kuzu
a little kuzu	a few chopped roasted nuts

1. Put the raisins in a pan with the salt and water to cover, and cook until soft. Add the apple and pear slices and simmer for 2 minutes. Thicken with a little kuzu dissolved in cold water. Transfer to 4 individual glass dishes.
2. To make the custard bring the soy milk to the boil and add the vanilla essence and the rice syrup. Thicken with a little kuzu dissolved in cold water. Pour over the fruit, garnish with a few chopped, roasted nuts and serve.

YIN ***Lemon Mousse*** ◎

SERVES 6–8

600ml (1 pint) Rice Dream Original
 rice milk
3 heaped dessertspoons agar agar
 flakes
a pinch of sea salt
2 dessertspoons kuzu or arrowroot

3–4 tablespoons lemon juice
2 tablespoons ground almonds *or*
 1 tablespoon tahini
3–4 tablespoons corn and barley
 malt syrup
a few lemon slices *or* roasted almonds

1. Place the Rice Dream in a saucepan and add the agar flakes. Soak for about 10 minutes to soften the agar. Place the pan on the heat and gently bring to the boil, stirring from time to time. Simmer for a few minutes until all the flakes have dissolved and then add a pinch of sea salt.
2. Dissolve the kuzu in 2 tablespoons cold water, then add this to the Rice Dream, stirring all the time until it thickens.
3. Remove from the heat and add the ground almonds or tahini, the corn and barley malt syrup and the lemon juice. Adjust the sweetness to your taste by adding a little more syrup or lemon juice, stir well and place the mousse in a wet, shallow bowl to cool for about an hour.
4. Place in a deep bowl or blender beaker and whisk with a hand blender for a few minutes to lighten the mousse and make it fluffy. The longer you blend and the more air you get into the mixture, the lighter it will be.

Spoon into 6–8 individual glass dishes and garnish with lemon slices or roasted almonds. This dessert keeps well in the refrigerator for 2–3 days.

VARIATION

Sweeten with apple and strawberry juice concentrate instead of rice syrup and blend in a few fresh strawberries instead of the lemon juice.

YANG   ## Apple Crumble

You can use different fruits according to the season.

SERVES 6–8

6 large eating apples, cored and sliced	175g (6oz) rolled oats
½ teaspoon ground cinnamon	50g (2oz) chopped walnuts
200ml (7fl oz) apple juice	100ml (4fl oz) rice syrup or barley malt
½ teaspoon sea salt	
1 heaped tablespoon kuzu	100ml (4fl oz) corn or sunflower oil
110g (4oz) wholewheat pastry flour	1 teaspoon vanilla essence

1. Preheat the oven to 190°C/375°F/Gas Mark 5.
2. Place the apples in a pan with the cinnamon, apple juice and a pinch of sea salt. Simmer for a few minutes, then dissolve the kuzu in cold water and stir into the fruit to thicken.
3. Mix together the flour and oats and dry-roast in a heavy pan for 5 minutes, stirring all the time. Mix in a bowl with the walnuts and salt. Blend the rice syrup or

malt, oil and vanilla separately and add to the dry ingredients.

4. Pour the fruit into an ovenproof dish and cover evenly with the crumble mix. Place in the preheated oven and cook for about 20 minutes or until golden brown on top. Allow to cool a little before serving.

YIN ## *Strawberry Couscous Cake*

This is quite a fiddly dish, but ideal for dinner parties and other celebrations.

SERVES 6–8

3 cups (600ml/1 pint) apple juice	2 cups (375g/13oz) couscous
2 tablespoons raisins	2 tablespoons tahini or almond butter
2 tablespoons ground almonds	(see Glossary)
a pinch of sea salt	black cherry sugar-free jam
1 teaspoon vanilla essence	toasted flaked almonds, sliced strawberries
1 teaspoon ground cinnamon	and lemon juice

1. Put the apple juice, raisins, ground almonds, salt, vanilla essence and cinnamon in a pan and bring to the boil. Add the couscous, remove from the heat and cover tightly. Leave unopened for 20 minutes.

2. Stir well, then press half the mixture into a wet mould (cake tin, spring mould or similar). Mix the tahini or almond butter with 2 tablespoons jam and beat into a cream. Spread this over the couscous mixture in the mould. Add the remaining couscous, pressing down

well with a wet spatula or the palm of your hand. Leave to stand for a while before turning on to a large plate.

3. Spread some jam around the sides of the cake and press on some flaked almonds to cover. If you have some jam left, spread some over the top of the cake. Now cover with sliced strawberries, sprinkle over the lemon juice and a few flaked almonds, and serve.

VARIATION

If you wish, you can make a simple glaze to top the cake with equal amounts of jam and hot water (you may want to try a lighter jam like apricot).

Baked Stuffed Apples

The lemon and syrup add a wonderfully tangy flavour to baked apples.

SERVES 4

4 large eating apples, cored	a few drops of lemon juice
1 tablespoon chopped nuts	a few drops of vanilla essence
1 tablespoon raisins	¼ teaspoon ground cinnamon
1 level teaspoon miso	1 tablespoon lemon juice
½ teaspoon grated lemon rind	1 tablespoon barley malt or rice syrup

1. Mix the nuts, raisins, miso, lemon rind, a few drops of lemon juice, vanilla essence and cinnamon together and press into the apples. Place them on a baking tray and bake in the oven at 180°C/350°F/Gas Mark 4 until just soft. Remove from the oven and cool a little.

2. Place the apples in individual serving bowls. Mix 1 tablespoon lemon juice and the malt or syrup together, drizzle over the top and serve.

BREAKFAST DISHES

Breakfast is often the most important meal for people who are out at work most of the day. Simple, light Vegetable Miso Soup (see page 87) is ideal, perhaps with a few noodles, steamed bread or some leftover grains. Some people enjoy a vegetable dish with a pickle accompaniment to start the day. Steamed or toasted sourdough bread can be used from time to time, with a spread like tahini, rice or barley malt, puréed apples or vegetables. Try Tahini and Lemon Dip (see page 134) or Carrot and Nut Dip (see page 135).

Or you can make delicious porridges from whole oats, rolled or jumbo oats or leftover grains like rice or millet. You can flavour your porridge with a selection of toasted seeds or nuts, Gomashio (see page 149), green nori flakes, or for sweetness try raisins, barley malt or a little amasake.

Drink can include Bancha Twig Tea (see page 148) or grain coffee. Try to use as much variety as possible and don't plan too far ahead – it is good to wake up in the morning not quite knowing what breakfast will be . . .

YANG *Whole Oat Porridge*

Great on a cold winter's morning.

SERVES 4

1 cup (175g/6oz) whole oats

a pinch of sea salt

1. Wash the oats and soak them in 6 cups (1.5 litres/2½ pints) water for 6 hours or overnight.
2. Place the oats in the pressure cooker with the salt and bring to pressure. Place over a flame diffuser, turn the heat down very low and cook for about 50 minutes.
3. Alternatively, cook very slowly in a covered cast iron pot on a flame diffuser for several hours, stirring from time to time.

Jumbo or Rolled Oat Porridge

Soaking the oats overnight before simmering gives a creamier, more digestible porridge.

SERVES 2

1 cup (110g/4oz) jumbo or rolled oats

a pinch of sea salt

1. Put the oats in a heavy pan with the salt and 2½–3 cups (600–850ml/1–1¼ pints) water. Bring to a simmer, stirring from time to time.
2. Place a flame diffuser under the pan, reduce the heat to very low, and cover. Simmer for 20–25 minutes, giving an occasional stir.

Rice Porridge

SERVES 4

1 cup (200g/7oz) brown rice
a pinch of sea salt

1. Wash the rice and drain thoroughly. Place in a heavy-based pan with 5 cups (1.25 litres/2¼ pints) cold water and salt. Cook, covered, for 50–60 minutes.

Leftover Grain Porridge

Generally take 1 cup (175g/6oz) ready-cooked rice, millet, barley or similar, place in a pan and barely cover with water. Simmer gently on a flame diffuser for about 20 minutes. The more you stir it, the creamier it will get.

Vegetable and Fruit Purées

Carrot, pumpkin or onion spread or purée can be easily made by gently cooking (together or separately) sliced vegetables in a little water with a pinch of sea salt until soft. Mash or blend until smooth. Sliced apples or pears make a nice sweet version – try adding a few raisins or sultanas before blending.

Bancha Twig Tea

Boil about 600ml (1 pint) water and add 1 level tablespoon bancha twigs. Simmer for about 5 minutes, strain and serve.

Fast boiling over long periods tends to make the tea bitter, so make sure you only boil for a short period. You can re-use the twigs, adding a few extra each time and boiling again.

CONDIMENTS

Roasted Dulse and Pumpkin Seed Condiment

This has a slightly nutty flavour.

25g (1oz) dulse
110g (4oz) pumpkin seeds

1. Check the dulse carefully for bits of shell but do not wash. Place on a tin tray and roast in the oven, at 180°C/350°F/Gas Mark 4, for just a few minutes until crunchy. Remove and grind thoroughly.
2. Wash and drain the pumpkin seeds and dry-roast in a frying pan until plump and golden, stirring gently all the time.
3. Grind the roasted pumpkin seeds with the dulse in a suribachi. Allow to cool before transferring to a sealed glass container. Use as needed on grains.

Gomashio (Sesame Salt)

20–24 teaspoons sesame seeds
1 teaspoon sea salt

1. Check the sesame seeds for stalks and stones. Wash and drain but do not allow to dry out.
2. Dry-roast the sea salt in a heavy pan for a few minutes, then grind in a suribachi. Dry-roast the seeds, stirring constantly for about 5–10 minutes. When done, the seeds will start to pop, giving off a nutty aroma and will crush easily between the thumb and finger.
3. Quickly add to the salt in the suribachi and grind slowly and evenly until half crushed – not to a fine powder. Cool and store in a glass container. Use on grains. Sesame salt will keep for several weeks but is best made fresh weekly.

Roasted Sunflower Seeds

It's a good idea to roast a batch to last a week or two and keep the seeds in a sealed jar, handy for regular use as snacks and garnishes.

1. Rinse the seeds in a wire sieve and drain thoroughly but do not dry. Heat a heavy-based frying pan and add the seeds. Stir with a wooden spoon or spatula to stop them burning. Keep stirring gently until the seeds are a golden brown colour all over.
2. Transfer to a dish to cool, then place in a glass jar and seal.

9

THE MACROBIOTIC LIFESTYLE

Eating natural food, prepared according to natural principles, is undoubtedly important for our health. But we really need to burn this 'fuel' in a productive fashion. It is little use sitting at home or in the office, eating delicious macrobiotic food but not engaging in physical activity, cleaning, self-reflection or contact with the external natural world. However, if you combine a 'macrobiotic lifestyle' with eating well-prepared macrobiotic food, then you are likely to experience a much quicker and more marked improvement in your level of vitality.

By engaging in the activities described in this chapter, you will speed up the elimination of toxins from your body. Even if you simply eat the food, without making any further effort, change will inevitably occur but more slowly; and you will probably lose patience. On the other hand, if you change your lifestyle as well as eating good-quality macrobiotic food, you can make a dramatic difference to your health and well-being.

None of these ideas are particularly new or unique – they are simply traditional wisdom. If you had the opportunity to consult your great-great-grandmother about making changes in your diet and lifestyle she would almost certainly make many of the suggestions listed below! In the absence of your great-great-grandmother, just recall or observe the habits of an elderly member of your family or community. They may not have eaten macrobiotic food but they will definitely have practised many of the suggestions that follow.

CHEWING WELL

Chewing your food well is a great help to your digestion. This is particularly true of any diet that is high in carbohydrate (in the case of macrobiotics this refers to the use of whole cereal grains and grain by-products). Meat and other animal by-products do not require as much saliva because they rely on the stronger acids of the lower part of the digestive tract. This is why dogs and other carnivores can simply bolt their food, knowing that their digestive system will take care of the process later on. But this is not the case with a diet high in carbohydrate.

On a sensory level, cereal grains taste sweeter and more delicious the longer you chew them. This is quite the opposite to chewing the same piece of meat for several minutes – it actually begins to taste worse! Ideally, you should chew each mouthful up to 30 times. This may sound a tall order initially. However, with time and practice, you will start to wonder how you ever enjoyed your food when you chewed each mouthful only 5–10 times. Chew slowly and wait until the food in your mouth has dissolved into liquid before you swallow.

It is also important to avoid distractions while you eat. Our contemporary culture makes it very hard to find the time to chew slowly and quietly, without the distractions of the telephone or the television. When we are mentally distracted while eating, the various organs that aid the digestive process later on (liver, gall bladder, stomach, pancreas and small intestine) are more likely to become more Yang and tense and therefore less efficient in aiding the digestive process. This can leave you feeling uncomfortable, irritable and bloated.

Try to avoid eating while you are standing or walking, and don't have meals during business meetings or while engaged in a telephone conversation. It would also be wise to avoid watching television, reading, writing or trying to do a crossword puzzle. Certainly the worst scenario would be eating while engaged in a serious argument! In an ideal world, the process of eating your food needs to be slow and peaceful, allowing you the opportunity to savour what you are eating and to reflect on how it was prepared. This also helps you develop an appreciation of the person who prepared it.

I believe that we can all benefit from 'chewing well' in

all aspects of life. It is rather like reading the small print on a legal document. When we rush anything our appreciation of it tends to be shallow and the benefits correspondingly superficial. Our contemporary lifestyle demands ever-increasing levels of speed and mental agility, and we expect our bodies to keep up with this pace. However, by chewing well in all areas of our life, we can benefit from a new-found sense of harmony and stability.

In addition, chewing anything well allows you to absorb and disseminate information more efficiently, which in turn helps you decide what you need and what you can discard. The same metaphor can be applied to this book – some of the ideas you will take to immediately, while others you may need to ponder and 'chew over' for longer. You may then absorb them into your lifestyle or reject them as inappropriate for you.

HAVING CONTACT WITH NATURE

By eating whole, natural macrobiotic foods you are already making a unique contact with nature. These foods have not been processed in a faceless industrialised plant but have had all the benefits of simple growing techniques and have been brought to your local shop with the minimum of fuss, packaging and processing. This direct contact with nature through your daily food inevitably leads to a greater concern for and awareness of the environment. You only have to enter your local natural food store and you will find leaflets and brochures on every aspect of the environment and our responsibility to protect it.

It can be extremely beneficial to mirror this 'internal' contact with nature by spending more time in the natural world. For instance, in warmer weather you could simply kick off your shoes for 10 minutes and walk barefoot on the grass. At weekends or in the evenings, make the effort to take a stroll in the woods, along a beach or in a nearby park. Try, as far as possible, to face the challenges that the weather may throw at you – really feel the cold, albeit for a short time. During hot weather again, only for short periods, feel the heat of the sun on your skin. Have a bracing walk when it is wet, stormy or excessively windy.

Our ancestors faced many of these challenges on a daily basis and, while we enjoy our modern comforts, they do distance and alienate us from the natural world. We can interact with nature through our daily food but experiencing the elements at first hand will greatly strengthen this contact.

TAKING EXERCISE

Imagine for a moment that you own a four-wheel drive vehicle. You can put the best fuel into the engine and keep it regularly serviced. But if you do not use it to its full capacity, and 'put it through its four-wheel drive paces' from time to time, it will inevitably seize up and begin to give you problems.

Human beings are much the same. The 'fuel' that we use in macrobiotics is the product of thousands of years of human evolution. Biologically speaking, it is our optimum fuel. Macrobiotic food is still based on a traditional Japanese farmer's diet. But, to gain maximum benefit from this special fuel, it is vital to take regular exercise.

If you are overweight, have a health problem or are taking medication or have not exercised regularly in recent months, you should always seek the advice of your medical practitioner before you undertake a regular exercise regime. Moderate the exercise suggestions that follow according to your age, level of fitness, blood pressure and whether or not you are overweight.

There is no one simple exercise routine that will be right for everybody. But here are some guidelines that you can use to design your own activity. Firstly, whatever exercise you choose to take on, make sure you do it regularly – at least three times a week. Secondly, you need to exercise for at least 20 minutes. Thirdly, if your fitness level allows, make your exercise vigorous enough to make you sweat and become breathless. The fourth and final criteria is that your exercise programme should be a bit of a challenge. Practically speaking, if your current level of fitness is poor, then simply walking 1.5–2.5km (1–1½ miles) to work three times a week would be enough of a new challenge for you to undertake. However, someone who is exceptionally fit would have to walk or run a longer distance in a shorter time.

Generating sweat and becoming breathless while you exercise both speed up the process of elimination. The main elimination organs are: the lungs, the kidneys, the liver and the large intestine. In Chinese medicine, the skin is regarded either as 'the third lung' or 'the third kidney' and is used as another channel of elimination. Similarly, stretching your lung capacity can strengthen your circulation and supply a rich source of oxygen to your blood which, apart from the physiological benefits, will also leave you feeling emotionally more positive and clear.

GETTING UP EARLY

Traditionally, our ancestors were always awake and active around sunrise. And this is also true of all the Third World countries that I have visited in the last 25 years. If this is a challenge to your current lifestyle, then at least make the effort for the next 30 days. In a four-season climate, it means getting up earlier in the summer and a little later in the winter. The Ki energy of sunrise provides the foundation on which your whole day is built. Miss out on this vital time of day by sleeping until 9 or 10 a.m. and you are bound to feel tired and unenthusiastic as the day progresses. The early part of the day supports the physiological function of the liver which in Chinese medicine strengthens our muscles, our flexibility and, on a Ki level, our creativity.

Once you are up and about in the morning, you should do some form of exercise or stretches (see pages 164–9) before you eat. It is also wise to wait until you are hungry before you have any breakfast. A common cause of feeling unenthusiastic first thing in the morning is having eaten too late the night before or having stayed up too long. For these first 30 days, try to be asleep before midnight and avoid eating for one to two hours before you go to bed.

ENJOYING REGULAR TOWEL RUBS

Since your skin is a major elimination organ – associated with the lungs and the kidneys – activating it strongly in the morning and evening will speed up the process of elimination. Simply brushing your skin briskly with a brush or a loofah is too superficial. This can help remove dead skin and the abrasive quality is known to encourage the immune system to kick in more strongly to repair the minor damage. However, I prefer a hot towel rub, as it not only stimulates the lympathic system but also improves your overall circulation.

Try to do this in the morning and the evening – soon after you rise and shortly before going to bed – for the next 30 days. Grasp a small hand towel at either end and dip the central portion, that you are not holding, into a basin of very hot water. Remove the towel from the water and wring it in opposite directions until it is almost dry.

Open up the towel and rub your skin vigorously all over your body, beginning with the face, neck, shoulders, arms, hands, fingers, the back, the front, the legs and finally the toes. Your skin should feel tingly and will perhaps turn pink. Pay particular attention to the extremities – the fingers and the toes – as this is where Ki energy enters and leaves the meridians of the body. Ki energy also has a habit of stagnating towards the extremities, especially in the webbing between the fingers and toes.

If you do not have enough time to have a regular towel rub or dislike the whole notion, then at least try to towel rub your feet and hands – especially between the fingers and toes in the morning and evening.

It is also important to regard this exercise as separate from towelling down after a shower or a bath. Remember that a bath or a shower is largely Yinising (relaxing), whereas a hot, vigorous towel rub is Yangising (stimulating).

AVOIDING LONG, HOT BATHS

A long, hot bath, although potentially relaxing, is actually very draining of your Ki and vital minerals. In Japan, very hot baths are popular but Japanese people's intake of salt from miso and shoyu is extremely high compared to other cultures. When you eat macrobiotically, your intake of salt from other sources – animal food in particular – is much, much lower and you will not have the reserves of salt. A short, hot bath or a short, hot shower is fine, as it is lingering for a long time which allows the leaching out of vital minerals and salts. If you insist on a daily hot bath, then:

♦ keep it short

♦ add a handful of sea salt to the water to help lessen your loss of vital minerals

Alternatively, at the end of a hot shower, give yourself a few seconds of cold water which helps to close up the skin pores and Yangise your overall condition. Similarly, in cultures that advocate saunas and Turkish baths, it is always traditional to Yangise at the end of these baths by plunging into cold water or taking a cold shower or rolling in the snow to help close the pores. It all comes back to Yin and Yang.

WEARING NATURAL FIBRE CLOTHING

Be very selective in the first 30 days of your practice of macrobiotics about what you wear close to your skin. The natural fibres of cotton or silk allow your skin to breathe adequately while at the same time preventing the build-up of any excessive electromagnetic charge. You can wear wool or other products provided they are not in direct contact with your skin. Practically speaking, this means buying socks, tights, stockings, underwear, vests, shirts, blouses and trousers that are either cotton or silk.

Since we spend up to a third of our day asleep, you should pay attention to the clothing that you wear in bed and of course the sheets and pillowcases. For many years I have been in favour of using the Japanese futon which is a 100 per cent layered mattress sewn in to a heavy-duty cotton shell. Traditionally these would be rolled up in the morning, regularly aired and replaced every year or two. Since they are relatively expensive, this may be impractical. But it is at least possible to air them, as cotton will absorb your sweat.

NURTURING PLANTS AT HOME

I have always been intrigued and fascinated by the Oriental tradition of bringing elements of the external world into our homes. Whether these were captive birds, ornamental fish tanks or exotic plants, they were designed to be a reminder of the world that we live in. Healthy plants in the home can provide an ionising effect on the atmosphere (especially the peace lily). They can also generate a feeling of uplifting Ki in the atmosphere and be a subliminal reminder to us all of the outside world.

Their health and vitality often reflects our own. In the Orient, there is a parallel between the breathing plant world and the function of our own lungs. If you live in a four-season climate, then I particularly recommend having a few delicate fern plants in your home, as they are reasonably easy to look after and provide an image of freshness and vitality when in good health.

SINGING

From my teacher and mentor, Michio Kushi, I learnt many years ago that whistling, singing, chanting and shouting are all natural expressions of Ki and can also provide another route for eliminating stagnant Ki from our systems. Think back ... When was the last time you had a really good shout or a sing-song? It is not unusual for these activities to give you a sense of release, relief and a new charge of energy.

For the past 100 years in England, men on football terraces have chanted, sung and shouted at their opponents or in support of their own team. Farm labourers and factory workers used to whistle and sing when they worked. And this tradition is still very much alive in most Third World countries.

So make the effort to sing a song every day at home, even if it's just singing along to your favourite CD track or to the radio while you are driving your car to work. Before dismissing the idea as totally non-you – give it a try and notice the difference!

CLEANING

Anyone initiating changes in their diet and lifestyle will benefit from living in a home that reflects their aspirations. From this perspective, we could argue that our inner world (our health) and our outer world (our environment) are completely interconnected. I am not suggesting that you should live in an antiseptic, highly polished vacuum but simply that you should have a close look at your home – especially your kitchen – and see what needs a good clean and what can be discarded.

I have always regarded cleaning on this level as a form of active meditation. When I began studying macrobiotics at the East West Centre in London in 1977, my first job was as a cleaner. For three hours every morning, I vigorously cleaned floors and stairways while reflecting on all the ideological and social issues that macrobiotics seems to have answers for. It was very grounding and also activated my Ki.

Similarly, a year later, when I undertook a committed study of shiatsu massage, I asked the teacher if I could have a discount or do some work in exchange. He gave me the job of cleaning and maintaining the dojo before and after class and I am convinced that it made me a more committed and attentive student. In Japan, for example, monks spend the early hours not in solitary meditation but in vigorous and silent cleaning of the monastery. And the few individuals I have met who had the opportunity to study with George Ohsawa have all commented that he was almost fanatical – even by Japanese standards – about cleaning and order. He always saw it as *his* task to keep his space clean and bright, rather than a student's or employee's responsibility.

Keep your windows clean and bright, as they are the eyes of your home and they allow a fresh charge of Ki to enter your space. Pay particular attention to your kitchen, especially if in recent weeks, months or years you have been cooking animal food. Get rid of all the grease and grime and, while you are cleaning the refrigerator and your cupboards, discard all the unwanted leftovers that you will no longer need because you are eating macrobiotic foods.

Your kitchen is the central point in your life for creating your blood and your future health, so it needs to reflect your vision. Clear out all the poisons from the dreaded 'cupboard under the sink' and replace them with environmentally friendly products which are widely available nowadays.

While you are in cleaning mode, get rid of any 'unwanted baggage' throughout your home. We all have accumulations of old clothes, books, notes, mementos, broken objects that we are going to fix one day, and bits and pieces that we think we may find useful in the future. Try to be ruthless and only surround yourself with those items that you love, and that are practical and useful at the moment.

ENGAGING IN SELF-REFLECTION

You may call this process meditation or prayer. But it's really just an opportunity to take a few moments of quiet and stillness every day to reflect on where you are, how you are, and what your next steps should be. In the hustle and bustle of daily life, it is very valuable to be still and at peace with yourself – even if it is only for a few minutes.

This process is very grounding and gives you the opportunity, when you begin macrobiotics, to check quietly on your own progress. Compared with our ancestors, we all live a very Yang, hectic and demanding life. Savouring a few moments of stillness, emptiness and Yin can provide a real haven from the stresses and strains of modern life. I would encourage you, however, to use the time creatively and think of ways that you can contribute to others and their lives, rather than becoming 'macroneurotic' and reflecting purely on your own needs.

If you find it difficult to sit still for a few minutes each day to meditate, try a more active form of self-reflection in the next section on Do-In.

PRACTISING DO-IN EXERCISES

The word 'Do' in Japanese has the same meaning and translation as the word 'Tao' in Chinese – the 'Path' or the 'Way'. It is frequently used in the Japanese language to describe various martial arts or spiritual disciplines, such as Kendo, Judo, Budo and Aikido. The word 'In' means 'at home'. In other words, practising a set of physical and spiritual exercises enables you to recharge your Ki energy and ground yourself but, most importantly, it allows your body's energy to self-regulate.

The following exercises are largely based on stretches of the meridians, specific pressure points along the meridians (acupressure), pounding the meridians with the fists, lightly brushing the meridians with the palm of the hands or tapping them with the fingertips. Do-In exercises also involve specific breathing techniques, meditation and chanting.

When I began macrobiotics I found the daily practice of Do-In particularly helpful in charging my energy, focusing my mind and reflecting on how my general condition appeared that day. I still practise it today. It is sometimes called the 'breakfast of the samurai', as it gives enormous flexibility, vitality and clear intuition.

To study this unique and fascinating system in more depth, consult *The Book of Do-In* by Michio Kushi (see Further Reading).

Good posture is vital to get the best results in Do-In exercises. Remember that Ki energy rises up through your feet, along the insides of the legs, up to the abdomen, out along the soft inner part of your arms, towards your fingertips, and across the surface of your face, leaving through the top of the head. This upward direction is known as the Yin and there are six Yin channels or meridians.

Conversely, Yang energy descends through the top of the head, down the back of the head, the back of the neck, the back, the back of the palms and the arms, through the lower back, the back and sides of the legs, and leaves through the toes. There are six of these Yang descending channels/meridians.

You can practise Do-In either standing, with your feet parallel and the same width apart as your hips; or you can sit comfortably in a chair with your back straight and your feet flat on the floor; or, if you prefer, you may sit in the Japanese seiza position (kneeling on the floor with your back straight and your feet tucked under your buttocks).

♦ Begin by raising your hands above your head while you look upwards towards the ceiling or sky. Do this by straightening, then relax your arms to your sides and bring your head down so that you are facing forward. You will find that your spine is now completely erect. Try to maintain this position throughout the exercises and always work barefoot or in cotton stockinged feet. (For the best results in warmer weather, practise the exercises outdoors or on the grass.)

♦ Spend a few moments centring your breathing. Begin by placing your tongue against the roof of your mouth and breathe in gently for 2–3 seconds through your nose, hold the breath for a further 2–3 seconds, and then breathe out for a further 3–4 seconds. Repeat this process for at least 2 minutes.

♦ The tools that you use in Do-In are your hands. Bring your hands together in prayer posture in front of you, at the height of your face, about 40cm (16 inches) ahead of you. While you press your hands firmly together, rub them vigorously at the same time, generating heat. Keep this up for 1–2 minutes, interspersing this vigorous rubbing with a few loud claps of the hands. Finish off by shaking your hands wildly to your sides, away from you, to help discharge old stagnant Ki from your system. You may now find that your hands feel very warm and tingly.

♦ With loose wrists and open palms, gently tap all over the top of your scalp. Again, with loose wrists, use your fingertips to rub your forehead and temples vigorously. Next, rub your cheeks up and down with the palms of your hands until they feel very warm and then shake out your hands to discharge the old Ki.

♦ Rotate your head in slow circles, breathing out as your head drops forward and breathing in as you rotate backwards. Repeat this exercise slowly several times and rotate your head in the opposite direction.

♦ With one of your arms stretched out to your side, and the palm facing forward, clench the fist of the other hand and, with the loose wrist, gently pound from the shoulder, along the soft part of the arm, to the fingertips. Then pound from the back of the hand, all the way back up to the shoulder. Repeat this 10 times on each arm and then shake out your hands briskly.

- ◆ Take a deep breath in and stretch your hands and arms as high as possible to your side, clench your fists and take a deep breath in. As you breathe out, pound the upper part of your chest with loose wrists but clenched fists, while exhaling through your nose. Repeat this exercise several times. For a more invigorating effect, you can give a lively 'Tarzan' yell at the same time!

- ◆ With your hands behind your back, clench your fists but keep them loose and pound your buttocks. This not only helps the movement of your Ki along the meridians of the back but also gets the blood to circulate that has become stagnant in the muscles of the buttocks.

- ◆ Rub your hands together, again at forehead height, slapping occasionally, and then shaking out your hands to replenish the Ki and discharge any stagnant energy.

- ◆ With loose wrists and tight fists, pound down the side of your legs towards your ankle and pound up the inside softer part of the legs inside. Repeat the exercise several times. However, you should avoid this exercise if you have any inflammation or varicose veins.

- ◆ Shake one of your feet vigorously from side to side, then kick forwards, kick sideways and try to kick backwards like a donkey. Repeat the exercise on the other leg.

- ◆ Without jumping up and down, just stamp your feet as quickly as possible on the floor for 30 seconds.

- Repeat this short set of exercises, sit comfortably either in a chair or in seiza posture, and bring your hands together in prayer position, arms together in front of your face. Narrow down your eyes so that they are almost closed. Repeat the breathing exercise as outlined at the beginning of this section and spend a few minutes peacefully putting your thoughts together for the day ahead.

10

WHERE TO GO FROM HERE

Whether you practise macrobiotics as a diet or a lifestyle or both, it is quite challenging to learn and apply it effectively in your life from a book alone. We tend to learn best from a teacher, a family member, or from the trial and error of working with a team. If you are keen to take your macrobiotic practice further, I therefore strongly recommend that your find out more about the system by reading other books, attending classes and cookery courses, or by being thoroughly spoilt at a macrobiotic summer camp or conference where you can learn and be catered for. There is an important social side of macrobiotics – discussing our practice, reviewing ideas, exchanging experiences and learning to take simple but effective short cuts as far as the cookery is concerned.

When I began my practice of macrobiotics, I seemed to spend half my day on cooking and, although I was fired up by the new ideas that I had discovered and new levels of energy that I was experiencing, the food seemed extremely bland. I tolerated it, because I believed there was no other option! But, after several months, I attended my first cookery course and went home with an enormous sense of relief and joy, having discovered that it did not need to take me so much time and that the food could taste absolutely delicious. On top of this, I discovered that there were others on the same path and I perhaps learnt more from their experiences than I did from the teacher.

Whatever route you choose to take with your practice of macrobiotics, I sincerely hope you will also discover new levels of energy, enthusiasm, creativity and curiosity. The single most important piece of advice I can give you on the journey is to chew well. Chew the food, chew the principles, and chew the ideas, to really absorb this fascinating system and gain the most benefit for your health, your family's health and for future generations.

FINDING MACROBIOTIC ADVICE AND SUPPORT

Worldwide, there are probably 50–75 macrobiotic consultants who have studied and practised the system for at least 15 years. The following contact points in the UK and USA are the best ways of finding well-trained, experienced practitioners. If you are still unclear about their background, be sure to ask them:

- ♦ Who did they study with?

- ♦ How long have they practised macrobiotics?

- ♦ Do they lecture, offer workshops, write books or have a clinic that they work from?

UK

The Macrobiotic Association of Great Britain, 377 Edgware Road, London W2 1BT
Tel: 07050 138419 Fax: 020 8741 0279
Email: *info@macrobiotic.co.uk*
Website: *www.macrobiotic.co.uk*

USA

The Kushi Institute, Box 7, Becket, MA 01223, USA
Website: *www.macrobiotics.org*
George Ohsawa Macrobiotic Foundation (GMOF)
Check the Macrobiotic Resources Network listed in their journal *Macrobiotics Today*, available from 1999, Myer Street, Oroville, CA 95966, USA

Europe

International Macrobiotic Assembly, Conscience Straat 44, B2018 Antwerp, Belgium
Email: *luc@owc.be*

What to Expect from a Consultation

Some individuals will have difficulty assessing whether their current condition is more Yin or more Yang. Or they may have other concerns about their health that make them feel they would benefit from an expert's advice.

Normally a consultation lasts one hour and the consultant uses Oriental diagnosis to assess through questioning, and perhaps examination of the hands, the eyes and the tongue, whether your condition is more Yin or more Yang and which organs are in need of support. They will normally question you on your current and past way of eating, your current symptoms and levels of fitness.

Generally most consultants will:

♦ Advise on what foods or aspects of your lifestyle you would be wise to leave alone for at least the next 30 days – perhaps longer.

♦ Give you clear dietary guidelines, including a list of ingredients and recipes for the preparation of all dishes including any special dishes, teas or condiments.

♦ Suggest adjustments in your lifestyle, including many of those described in Chapter 9 of this book.

They will normally recommend that you attend a cooking class and return for a follow-up consultation in approximately 30 days' time. At this point, they will reassess your condition and, if you are confident and feeling well, they will give you broader guidelines to follow for the months ahead. Most consultants do not require frequent follow-up visits unless you have a specific health problem.

Charges in the UK range between £30 and £60 for a consultation and in the USA from $150 to $250. Some macrobiotic consultants offer a reduced fee for any subsequent or follow-up consultations within a 12-month period.

GLOSSARY

agar agar (aygar) Jelling agent made from sea vegetables
almond butter A nut butter made from ground roasted almonds used for spreads or to enrich sauces or dressings
amazake Sweet, fermented preparation usually made from rice
arame Shredded sea vegetable
arrowroot Tropical root starch for thickening (use instead of kuzu)

bancha Sometimes called kukicha – roasted twig tea
barley malt Fermented grain sweetener

collards American term for spring greens

daikon (also mooli) Long, Chinese white radish
dulse Maroon-coloured sea vegetable from UK and USA

genmai miso Seasoning made from fermented rice, soya beans and sea salt

hatcho miso As genmai miso but contains no rice

hazelnut butter A nut butter made from hazelnuts – use as almond butter

hiziki Coarsely shredded sea vegetable, extremely rich in calcium

hummus Eastern Mediterranean pâté with chickpeas as main ingredient

Irish moss Sea vegetable also known as carragheen. Traditional Irish remedy ingredient

kanten Japanese jelly, savoury or sweet, made with agar flakes

kasha North European grain dish – usually buckwheat

kelp Local name for kombu, sea vegetable

koji A preparation used in fermentation of amazake, miso, etc.

kombu As for kelp – useful flavour enhancer and for softening dried beans

kukicha Roasted twig tea as bancha

kuzu Thickener prepared from Japanese mountain vine root. Very useful home remedy ingredient

laver Local name (Welsh) for nori, sea vegetable

millet Small, hard, yellow wholegrain

mirin Sweet rice cooking wine

miso Fermented soya bean seasoning – see genmai, hatcho, mugi, white

mochi Dried, pounded sweet ricecakes

mooli See daikon

mugi cha Roasted barley tea
mugi miso Fermented soya bean seasoning with barley
mugwort Herb used in flavouring grains such as mochi
mu tea Special strengthening tea created by George Ohsawa. Made from 16 different herbs including liquorice, cinnamon, ginger, ginseng

natto Fermented soya bean preparation usually purchased frozen from Japanese food shops – watch out for sugar and msg in the accompanying sauce!
natto miso chutney A delicious chutney made from soya beans, kombu, miso and ginger
nigari Sea salt by-product used to coagulate soya milk for tofu
nishime Special cooking style – steaming in heavy pot with kombu at the base. Very strengthening and delicious
nori Sea vegetable usually purchased in sheets and used toasted as a garnish or for wrapping sushi

oats Grain of European origin: whole form known as groats – excellent for winter porridge; jumbo – partially processed and steel cut; rolled or porridge oats are usually less nutritious than the above and cook much quicker

peanut butter Nut butter used for spreads and to enrich sauces etc. Watch out for added ingredients such as palm oil and sugar

quinoa (keenwah) Principal grain of the Incas. More protein than most grains, including rice. Nutty, nutritious and high in calcium and amino acids

177

🌀 **ramen** Quick noodle preparation usually with accompanying soup stock. Japanese versions of good quality are available in good wholefood stores

rice Principal grain for most areas of the Far East but also grown in USA and Europe. Essential staple for macrobiotic cooking

rice syrup Fermented sweet syrup made from rice

rutabaga American name for swede

sauerkraut Fermented cabbage, North European origin. The best ones are organic, salt and additive free

scallion American name for spring onions

sea salt The best are naturally harvested from the sea shore. Superior to most mined salts

seitan (saytan) High-protein food made from wheat gluten. Sometimes known as wheatmeat or gluten

shiitake Slow-growing mushroom which can be used dry or fresh. Good for stock and broth-making and also medicinally

shiso Red leaf used to produce colour in umeboshi pickling

shiso powder A condiment made from ground shiso leaves which is both salty and piquant

shoyu Naturally brewed soy sauce made from soya beans, wheat, salt and water

soba Japanese noodle available in several forms including 100 per cent buckwheat or 40 per cent buckwheat with wheatflour

somen Japanese wheat noodle – very thin

sourdough Usually fermented wheat starter used to prepare yeast-free, sourdough breads

soya milk Vegetable milk produced from white soya beans

sprout Vegetable seed which has been sprouted for use in salads

stoneground Traditional milling process for flour. Stone grinders retain more nutrients

suribachi Traditional Japanese grinding vessel with ridged sides to trap seeds. Used for mixing, grinding and puréeing. The wooden grinding tool is called a surikogi

sushi General a rolled rice preparation with nori, seasonings, pickles and vegetables or fish

sushi mat Useful bamboo mat for rolling sushi and for covering food

sweet rice Sticky, glutinous rice used for mochi and rich grain dishes. Check that it does not contain sugar or glucose

tahini Sesame seed paste

tekkuan Long-term pickled daikon. Strong flavour with salt and rice bran

tamari Traditional, natural-brewed soy sauce without wheat

tekka A very strong, salty condiment based on long-cooked vegetables

tempeh Versatile fermented soya bean preparation, usually bought frozen. Unlike tofu which can be served raw on occasions, tempeh has to be cooked

tempura Rich cooking style where food is dipped in batter and deep-fried

tofu Far Eastern soya bean 'cake' bought fresh and used in a wide variety of dishes. Made from soya beans and coagulated with nigari. Not fermented

udon Japanese noodle usually wholewheat but sometimes with rice flour added

umeboshi traditional Japanese pickle made from sour plums, shiso leaves and sea salt. Useful flavouring and home remedy ingredient. Avoid those in Japanese shops which include colours, sweeteners and preservatives

ume su Sometimes called umeboshi vinegar or red plum seasoning. Salty and sour red liquid used for dressings and seasoning

wakame Sea vegetable. Useful for soups and salads

wasabi Japanese horseradish powder with highly pungent flavour. Avoid those with colours and sweeteners

white miso Delicate, sweet and mellow miso preparation ideal for emphasising sweetness in root vegetable stews and summer soups

whole grains Any grain which is in its whole, original or slightly hulled form. Not flour, cracked or cut grain products

yannoh Roasted cereal grain coffee drink

FURTHER READING

MACROBIOTICS AND COOKERY

Aveline Kushi, *Complete Guide to Macrobiotic Cooking*, Warner Books, 1985

Kristina Turner, *The Self-Healing Cookbook*, Earth Tones Press, 1987

Michio Kushi, *The Book of Macrobiotics*, Japan Publications, 1987

Michio Kushi, *Holistic Health Through Macrobiotics*, Japan Publications, 1993

Herman Aihara, *Basic Macrobiotics*, Japan Publications, 1985

Jon Sandifer, *The 10-Day Re-Balance Programme*, Rider Books, 1997

MACROBIOTIC LIFESTYLE

Lino Stanchich, *Power Eating Program*, Healthy Products Inc., 1989

Denny Waxman, *Ten Steps to Strengthening Health*, Strengthening Health Publishing, 1997

Michio Kushi, *The Book of Do-In*, Japan Publications, 1979

Jon Sandifer, *Acupressure*, Element Books, 1997

USEFUL ADDRESSES

The Macrobiotic Association of Great Britain, 377 Edgware Road, London W2 1BT
Tel: 07050 138419 Fax: 020 8741 0279 Website: *www.macrobiotic.co.uk* Email: *info@macrobiotic.co.uk*
The Macrobiotic Association of Great Britain is a non-profit-making organisation set up in 1995 to provide a network for the macrobiotic community. They offer a bi-monthly journal, monthly luncheons and a useful resource pack for further information on macrobiotics in Great Britain.

One Peaceful World Society, PO Box 10, Becket, MA 01223, USA
Tel: (413) 623 2322 Email: *opw@macrobiotics.org*
OPW is an international macrobiotic information network and society founded in 1986 by Michio Kushi. The OPW publishes the quarterly OPW journal, One

Peaceful World Press and Macrobiotics Online – an internet site with the Kushi Institute.

George Ohsawa Macrobiotic Foundation, 1999 Myers Street, Oroville, CA 95966, USA
Tel: (530) 533 7702 Fax: (530) 533 7908 Email: *foundation@gomf.macrobiotic.net* GOMF is the publisher of the excellent bi-monthly journal *Macrobiotics Today*. They also offer discounts on book purchases and tuition on their annual French Meadows Summer Camp. Their website is: *www.gomf.macrobiotic.net*

SHOPS

Bumble Bee Natural Foods, 30 Brecknock Road, London N6 0DD. Tel: 020 7607 1936

Bushwacker Whole Foods, 132 King Street, Hammersmith, London W6 0QU. Tel: 020 8748 2061

Fresh & Wild, 196 Old Street, London EC1V 9FR. Tel: 020 7250 1708 Website: www.freshandwild.com

Fresh & Wild, 49 Parkway, Camden Town, London NW1 7PN. Tel: 020 7428 7575

Fresh & Wild, 210 Westbourne Grove, London W11 2RH. Tel: 020 7229 1063

Fresh & Wild, 305–311 Lavender Hill, London SW11. Opening October 2000.

Fresh & Wild, 71–75 Brewer Street, London W1. @ Opening December 2000.

Pauls Soyfoods Ltd. Delivers tofu, bread and organic produce. Tel: 01664 60572 Fax: 01664 410345

Planet Organic, 42 Westbourne Grove, London W2 5SH. Tel: 020 7221 7171

Loaves and Fishes, 52 The Thoroughfare, Woodbridge, Suffolk IP12 1AL. Tel: 01394 385650

Seasons, 8 Well Street, Exeter. Tel: 01392 436125

Clear Spring Direct, 19a Acton Park Estate, The Vale, London W3 7QE. Tel: 020 8746 0152. Fax: 020 8811 8893. Email: *mailorder@clearspring.co.uk* Website: *www.clear-spring.co.uk* (online shopping).

MACROBIOTIC COOKERY COURSES

Bob Lloyd, 99 Yeldham Road, Hammersmith, London W6 8JQ. Tel/Fax: 020 8741 0279. Email: *boblloyd@macrobiotic.co.uk*

Montse Bradford, The Natural Cookery School, Greenfields, Lovington, Castle Cary, Somerset BA7 7PX. Tel: 01963 240641 Website: www.montsebradford.com

The Concord Institute, 14 Blackstock Mews, Blackstock Road, London N4 2BT. Tel: 020 7359 6040

Check with the Macrobiotic Association of Great Britain for a more complete, current list.

HOLIDAYS AND SUMMER CAMPS

Macrobiotic Summer Camp and Conference, 3 Hamsey Close, Brighton, East Sussex BN2 5GQ. Tel: 01273 279439

Vegi Ventures, Castle Cottage, Castle Acre, Norfolk PE32 2AJ.

Kushi Institute Summer Conference, Box 390, Becket, MA 01223 USA

George Ohsawa Macrobiotic Foundation Camp, PO Box 426, Oroville, CA 95965, USA

Fall Health Classic, PO Box 30254, Santa Barbara, CA 93139-0254, USA

Pacific Macrobiotic Conference Tel: (510) 559 8057 Website: *www.alchemycalpages.com*

WORKSHOPS WITH JON SANDIFER AND BOB LLOYD

A one-day workshop offering a unique opportunity to acquire a grounding in the principles of macrobiotics, Oriental diagnosis and macrobiotic cookery. It is designed for beginners and runs from 10 a.m. until 4 p.m. The topics covered include:

* Discussion on macrobiotic food and cookery

* A macrobiotic cookery demonstration

* A macrobiotic lunch

* What is macrobiotics?

* Yin and Yang and our health (Oriental diagnosis)

* Personalised health advice from Jon Sandifer

* Questions and answers

For further details, please contact Bob Lloyd, 99 Yeldham Road, London W6 8JQ. Tel/Fax: 020 8741 0279 Email: *boblloyd@macrobiotic.co.uk*

THE 10-DAY RE-BALANCE PROGRAMME WITH JON SANDIFER

This is a 10-day residential course held annually in Switzerland, the USA and Great Britain, led by Jon Sandifer. It covers all the Yin/Yang principles for assessing your condition, cooking classes, Feng Shui, Do-In exercises and much, much more. For further details, please contact
Jon Sandifer, PO Box 69, Teddington, Middlesex TW11 9SH. Tel/Fax: 020 8977 8988.
Email: *jonsandifer@compuserve.com*
Website: *www.jonsandifer.com*

GENERAL INDEX

Note: Page numbers in *italics* refer to the Glossary.

FOOD AND RECIPE INDEX

Note: Page numbers in **bold** refer to recipes, numbers in *italics* refer to the Glossary.

PIATKUS BOOKS

If you have enjoyed reading this book, you may be interested in other titles published by Piatkus. These include:

Ambika's Guide to Healing and Wholeness: The energetic path to the chakras and colour Ambika Wauters

Ask Your Angels: A practical guide to working with angels to enrich your life Alma Daniel, Timothy Wyllie and Andrew Ramer

Barefoot Doctor's Handbook for the Urban Warrior: A spiritual survival guide Barefoot Doctor

Chakras: A new approach to healing your life Ruth White

Channelling for Everyone: A safe, step-by-step guide to developing your intuition and psychic abilities Tony Neate

Chinese Elemental Astrology: How the five elements and your animal sign influence your life EA Crawford and Teresa Kennedy

Chinese Face and Hand Reading Joanne O'Brien

Clear your Clutter With Feng Shui Karen Kingston

Colour Healing Manual: The complete colour therapy programme Pauline Wills

Creating Sacred Space With Feng Shui Karen Kingston

Energy Medicine: How to use your body's energies for optimum health and vitality Donna Eden with David Feinstein

Feng Shui Astrology: Using 9 star ki to achieve harmony and happiness in your life Jon Sandifer

Feng Shui Kit, The: The Chinese way to health, wealth and happiness at home and at work Man-Ho Kwok

Feng Shui Journey: Achieving health and happiness through your

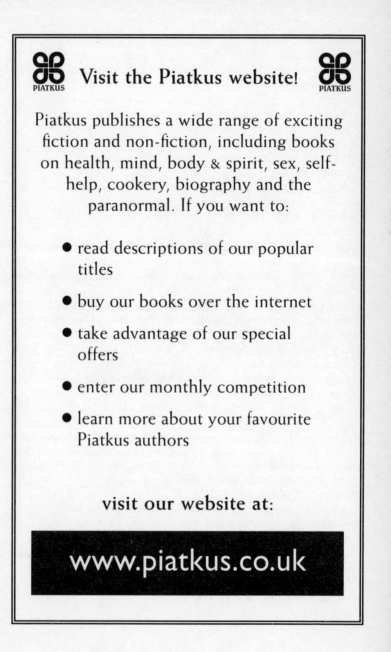